Fatty Liver Diet

85 Step-by-Step Recipes and Guide To Reverse Fatty Liver Disease And Live Longer

MELODY AMBERS

ISBN- 9781798705186

DEDICATION

To my three best friends; Ruth, Amy and Chloe;
You make cooking fun!

TABLE OF CONTENTS

Other Books By Melody Ambers

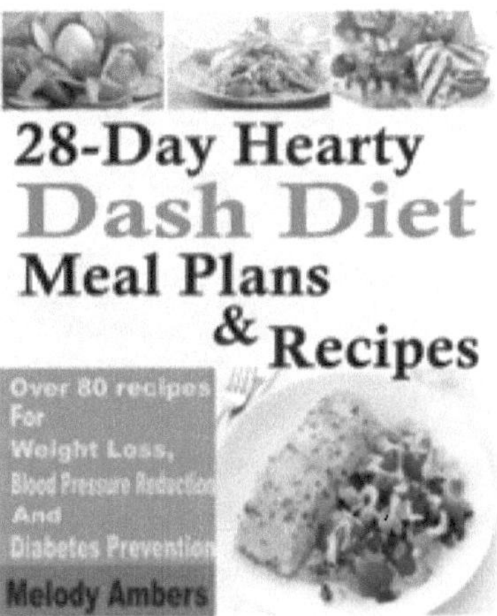

28-Day Hearty Dash Diet Meal Plans & Recipes: Over 80 recipes For Weight Loss, Blood Pressure Reduction And Diabetes Prevention

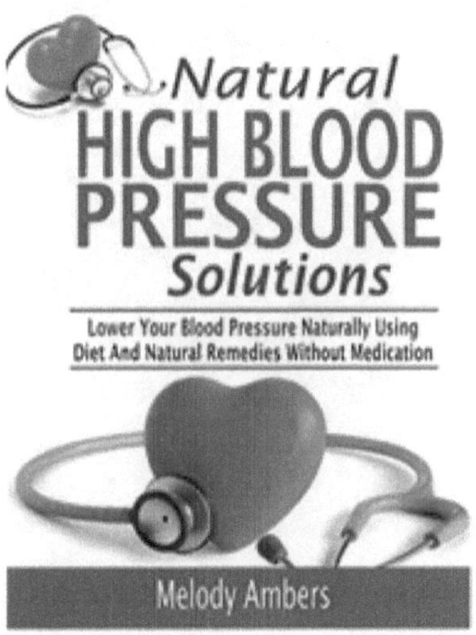

Natural High Blood Pressure Solutions: Lower Your Blood Pressure Naturally Using Diet And Natural Remedies Without Medication

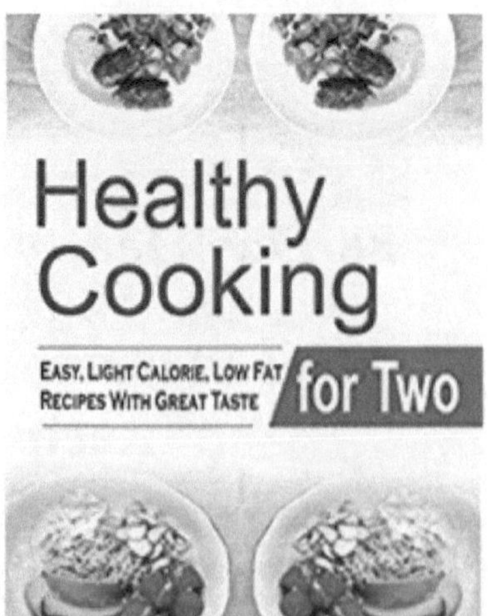

Healthy Cooking For Two: Easy, Light Calorie, Low Fat Recipes With Great Taste

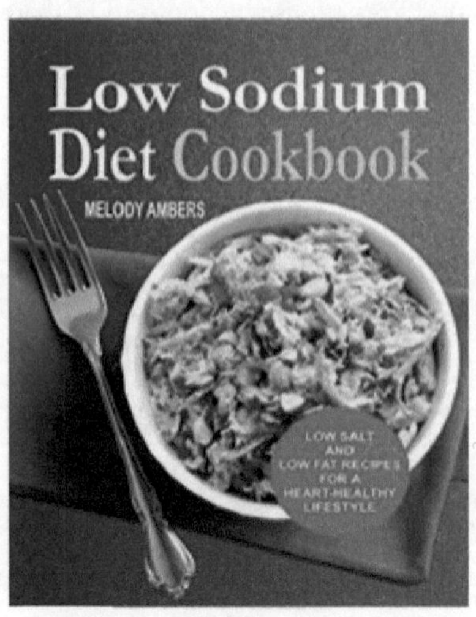

Low Sodium Diet Cookbook: Low Salt And Low Fat Recipes For A Heart-Healthy Lifestyle

INTRODUCTION

An Overview Of Fatty Liver Disease

The liver is the largest organ in the body. It performs very important tasks, acting as a support organ to many other organs of the body. It helps the body to digest food, remove poison from the blood and process our waste. The liver processes dietary fat and blood fat. Therefore, it is quite normal for it to have a bit of fat from time to time. However, if the fats start to build up, then you have a condition commonly known as fatty liver disease, in its simple form. However, if this condition is not reversed, then the fatty liver could deteriorate to inflammation, liver damage and liver cancer.

We have a responsibility to keep our liver healthy and clean, if we want it to work well and be free of complications. We need a healthy liver to survive. Fatty liver, a condition of excess fat storage in the liver, is the most common problem for the liver and sadly, a silent health crisis that affects a very large number of people in the world.

There are two types of fatty liver:

- Nonalcoholic fatty liver disease (NAFLD)
- Alcoholic fatty liver disease (alcoholic steatohepatitis)

Nonalcoholic Fatty Liver Disease (NAFLD)

NAFLD is fatty liver disease that's not caused by alcohol intake. But it's even more worrisome, as it affects one third of the American adult population. As a matter of fact, it affects about 25% of people in the world, including more than 6 million children, (especially Asian and Hispanic children). It is the most common serious and long-term liver condition in the world. It may interest you to note that NAFLD is not caused by eating a high-fat diet. Rather, it is usually caused by persistently insulin resistance and high blood sugar. Most people who are overweight are prone to this disease. So are those with Type 2 diabetes or pre-diabetes and high blood pressure (hypertension). With the increasing rate of obesity, high cholesterol and type 2 diabetes in the United States, it is not a surprise that the rate of NAFLD is also on the increase.

Others who are at risk of having fatty liver also includes those who have hepatitis B or C; take certain medications; smoke or have been exposed to toxins; a poor diet with little exercise; as well as those who have undergone very rapid weight loss. Additionally, fatty liver disease is usually accompanied with other risk factors for heart disease such as high triglycerides. This is why people with fatty liver are much more likely to die of heart disease than of liver disease.

Alcoholic Fatty Liver Disease

Alcoholic fatty liver disease comes as a result of excessive alcohol consumption. When you drink alcohol, the liver goes to work by breaking most of it down, so that it can be flushed out from your body. But in the course of breaking it down, harmful substances may be generated. These substances can promote inflammation, damage the liver cells. The more alcohol you take, the more you damage your liver. This could lead to alcoholic hepatitis and cirrhosis (liver scarring)

Symptoms & Diagnosis Of Fatty Liver

At the early stages, a fatty liver can be free of inflammation. Therefore, those who have it may experience a few symptoms such as:

- Nausea
- loss of appetite
- weakness

- Gallstones
- Red itchy eyes
- Spider-like blood vessels
- Overheating of the body
- Edema (swelling of the legs)
- Weight excess in the abdominal area
- Excessive sweating

If the fatty liver is not reversed, after a while, it may lead to inflammation causing scarring (fibrosis). It can also progress to cirrhosis, a chronic, progressive life-threatening condition. This second stage of fatty liver disease is also known as Non-Alcohol Related Steatohepatitis (NASH).

Therefore you must see a doctor without delay if you have any of these persistent signs and symptoms:

- Jaundice
- Dark urine
- Itching skin
- Bruising easily
- Dark black tarry faeces (melena)
- Confusion or poor memory
- Swelling of the lower tummy area (ascites)

Diagnosis

Most people find out that they have fatty liver after undergoing a routine blood sample (liver function tests) for other reasons unrelated to fatty liver. Once the results indicates some abnormality, your doctor will then probe into your background, asking questions about your lifestyle, the drugs you take, supplements, diets, exercises you engage it, and the amount of alcohol you take.

Nevertheless, even with these questions, fatty liver disease is only confirmed by further tests such as a CT or CAT Scan or MRI scan, Ultrasound or FibroScan. Sometimes, it may be necessary to do a liver biopsy.

Reversing Fatty Liver

Fatty liver warns you of bigger trouble ahead. The good news is that you can do something about the fatty liver by simply making a few adjustments in diet and lifestyle.

FOR YOUR DIET:

<u>Reduce Sugar Intake And Other Refined Carbohydrates</u>

Foods high in carbohydrates are easy to digest and are immediately converted to blood sugar. Simple carbs, sugar and refined flours raise blood sugar and insulin levels chronically and also increase fat deposits in the liver. As a result, insulin, a fat- storing hormone, is released from the pancreas to clear out the blood sugar from the blood to the cells. However, a continuous release of insulin to deal with the influx of sugar will cause the cells to become resistant to its effects. This leads to diabetes, which causes fatty liver.

To reverse fatty liver, the insulin levels in the body must go down. Once you limit sugary and starchy foods, you will be able to lower your blood sugar levels and lower the amount of insulin your body calls for. Avoid sugary foods and food made with white flours. Limit whole grains carbs as well. Limit your consumption of bread, cereal, pasta, rice, cake, pastry, and snacks made with flour.

Avoid sugar and foods that contain added sugar. Also, you will need to lower your intake of grains and cereals (rye, wheat, barley, oats and corn), and starchy veggies such as potatoes.

Eat Healthy Fats

Eat foods that are high in monounsaturated fats. These include avocados, flaxseeds, raw nuts and mega-3 fats that can be found in fish. Healthy fats will nourish your body. Include such healthy fats like extra virgin olive oil, cold pressed coconut and cold pressed macadamia oil in your diet. Steer clear of deep fried food, preserved meat, extremely fatty meat, margarine, cheap cooking oil and partially

Eat Lots Of Raw Plant Food (Vegetables)

The most powerful liver healing foods are raw vegetables and fruits. They assist in cleansing and repairing the liver filter, so that it can do its work of trapping and removing fat and toxins from the bloodstream more effectively.

Eat plenty of vegetables in salad forms and even cooked vegetables too. Ensure you eat at least seven servings of vegetables each day (raw and cooked). Fruits are also good for the liver, but do not exceed two servings a day, especially if you have high blood sugar or insulin.

Broccolis, collards, kale, arugula, Brussels sprouts, daikon radish are all great foods that help to repair and heal your liver. Let your diet include garlic and onions as well, because they contain sulfur, which is a wonderful detoxifier

<u>**Eat More Protein**</u>

Protein is safe. It does not affect your blood sugar or insulin levels negatively. It also helps to reduce hunger and cravings, making it easier to eat less and lose weight. Good protein sources include poultry, fish, egg, legumes, low-fat diary and lean red meat. It is important to get your protein from healthy sources, such as free range or organic. Fish (Fresh and canned fish) are another excellent source. But, do not eat smoked or fried fish. Certain cheeses like parmesan, feta, ricotta and cottage are rich in protein that helps fight fatty liver. Whey protein powder is a rich protein source.

Drink Less Alcohol

Of course, you'll have to reduce your intake of alcohol or stop completely. Excess alcohol consumption has been proven to the second major cause of fatty liver. It causes inflammation and damages the liver cells, resulting in fatty liver. If you have fatty liver, it is advisable to limit your alcohol intake to one drink per day and abstain for 2 to 3 days before taking your next one drink.

To avoid fatty liver, men shouldn't drink more than 4 units of alcohol in a day while women shouldn't drink more than 3 units in a day (One unit being about 10 ml of pure alcohol).

PHYSICALLY:

<u>Lose Weight:</u> Weight loss is very important to reverse fatty liver. So if obese, consider losing weight. Even a 5% reduction of your body weight may be enough to lessen current and future accumulation of fats in the liver; but a weight loss of up to 10% is required to address more serious symptoms like liver inflammation. Nevertheless, it is better to lose a modest amount of weight and sustain it, than to lose a large amount and regain it later. Additionally, if you lose weight too fast, you could worsen your NAFLD. Weight loss should be a gradual process to avoid complications. Try to lose between 450 to 900 g (i.e. 1 to 2 lbs) in a week. Maintain a healthy weight by maintaining a good diet. Steer clear of diet supplements or fad diets.

<u>Exercise Regularly</u>

Regular exercises have been proven to be a very effective way of reversing fatty liver. Physical exercise improves insulin sensitivity, consequently reducing cholesterol production in the liver as well as its level in the blood. The most effective type of exercise is the endurance type such as resistant training and high intensity interval training (HIIT). Resistant training with the help of body weight or weight machines as well as exercises that increase heart rate such as jogging or brisk walking melt away surplus calories and aids effective weight loss. Aerobic exercises are best suited to burn off fat. Nevertheless, physical exercises have been confirmed to be very crucial to reversing fatty liver, irrespective of whether weight loss occurs or not.

Therefore, start by doing some physical activity, if you currently do not. Be active on most days of the week. Aim for a balanced exercise. Balance cardiovascular exercise such as jogging, cycling and walking with strength training using weights, or your own body weight. Aim to get some cardiovascular exercise every day or every other day, but ensure that you get some strength training once in a week.

Aim for 150 minutes (2½ hours) of reasonable intensity physical activity or 75 minutes (1¼hours) of vigorous intensity physical activity each week. You can even combine both moderate and vigorous activities, doing an equivalent of both.

You can get rid of the fat in your liver through regular exercises carried out several times a week. Your success will depend on the sustenance of the exercise that you do; and not just its intensity. However, always consult your doctor before starting a new exercise program.

Recipes To Reverse Fatty Liver

BREAKFAST RECIPES

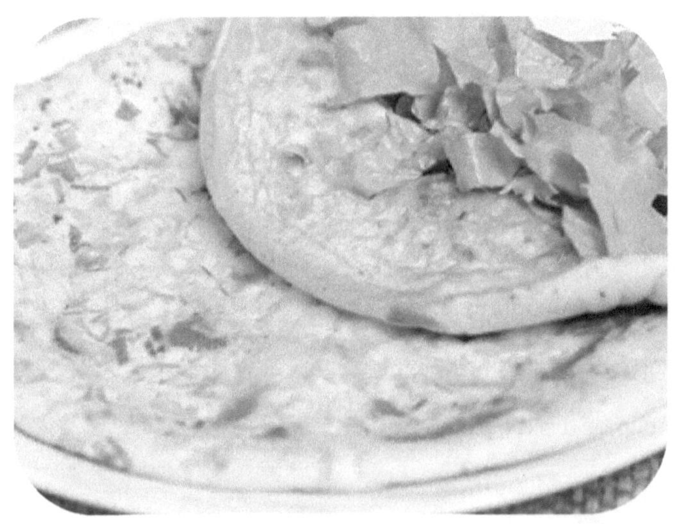

Chinese Vegetable Omelet

Start your morning with this quick, nutritious meal packed with vitamins C & K, which help to combat liver disease.

Preparation time: 3 minutes

Cooking time: 5 minute

Servings: 1

Ingredients:

2 eggs

1 tbsp low fat sour cream, creme fraiche or heavy cream

¼ cup of chopped green onion

1 tsp of minced garlic

¼ cup of diced tomato

¼ cup of chopped kale

Additions (All optional):

¼ cup of chopped bell pepper

1/8 cup of diced Serrano pepper

¼ cup of diced mushroom

Directions:

1. Whisk together the eggs and sour cream until fluffy. In a non-stick pan, lightly sauté the garlic, kale, tomato and onion, together with the optional ingredients over medium heat for about 3 minutes until softened.

3. Now add the whisked egg, cooking for up to 3 minutes until omelet can be lifted easily with a spatula.

4. Flip omelet and cook an additional minute.

5. Finally fold in half and cook per side for 30 more seconds. *Enjoy!*

Almond Crusted French Toast

A rich, hearty breakfast that's low in vitamin A, which is good for people with cirrhosis. It also contains loads of protein that your body needs.

Preparation time: 10 minutes

Cooking time: 15-17 minute

Servings: 6

Ingredients:

1½ cup (2%) milk

6 eggs

1 ½ tsp vanilla extract

4 tbsp honey

2 tsp salt

1 tsp orange zest

1 loaf of day old bread (brioche, challah, or baquette), sliced

½ cup slivered almonds

1 tablespoon butter

Optional Garnish:

Fresh berries

Powdered sugar

Squeeze of orange juice

Directions:

1. Whisk eggs, milk, honey, vanilla, salt and orange zest together.

2. Place the slices of bread in a shallow baking pan and pour mixture over evenly. Let it soak 2 minutes per-side.

3. Preheat a medium large skillet. Melt butter in it and dip a side of each bread slice in slivered almonds to coat well.

4. Add slices to pan in batches.

5. Sauté each side 3-4 minutes, until golden brown, and remove to a pan in the oven.

6. Once ready to eat, top with optional garnishes.

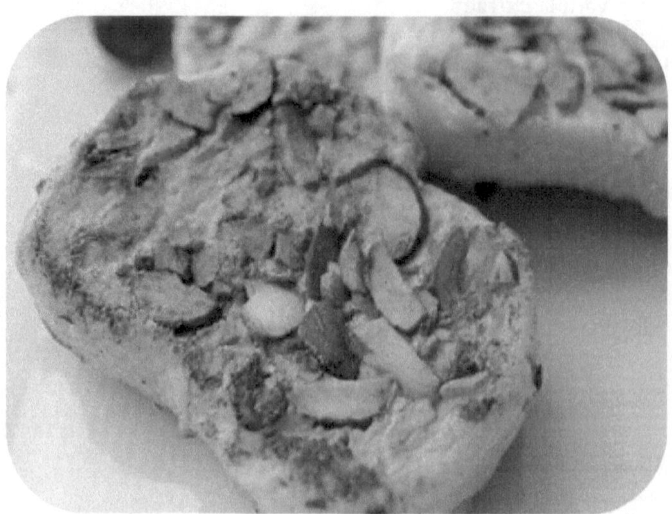

Liver –Friendly Corn Bread

Honey in this recipe help to control blood sugar levels which ultimately helps those who are at risk of fatty liver disease. Honey is loaded with good bacteria, and lots of good bacteria protect the liver from injury.

Preparation time: 10 minutes

Cooking time: 25minutes

Servings: 9

Ingredients:

1cup flour (gluten- free)

1/4 cup honey

3/4 cup yellow corn meal

1 cup almond milk

2tsp baking powder

1/4 cup coconut oil

1 egg, whole

Directions:

1. Preheat oven to 400°F. Grease an 8" pan with oil, preferably avocado.

2. Combine all the dry ingredients in a bowl.

3. Combine all the liquid ingredients in another bowl and then pour into the dry mix and stir until thoroughly incorporated.

4. Pour batter in pan and bake until golden brown.

Quick N Tasty Sunrise Oatmeal

Preparation time: 0 minutes

Cooking time: 5minute

Servings: 2

Ingredients:

1 cup of oat

1 cup of water

1 cup of milk or 2 cups of milk, to make it tastier

 3/4 cups blueberries, frozen

½ cup sour cherries, frozen

½ cup strawberries, frozen

2 tablespoons coconut flakes

1 tablespoons raw honey

Directions:

1. Add the milk and water to a pot and after 2-3 minutes; add the oat flakes, stirring constantly.

2. Once it starts to boil, stir another 3 minutes and then add the frozen fruit. Keep stirring on medium heat until mixture is dark red in color.

3. Remove to a bowl; add the honey and the coconut flakes and stir. *Enjoy!*

Berry Choc Breakfast Smoothie

Preparation time: 5minutes

Cooking time: minute

Servings: 2

Ingredients:

2 tablespoons goji berries, soaked overnight in water

3 tablespoons whey protein powder

1 tablespoon cocoa powder or cacao

1.5 cups milk of choice

1 tablespoon almond butter

Directions:

1. Add all ingredients to blender and blend to desired smoothness.

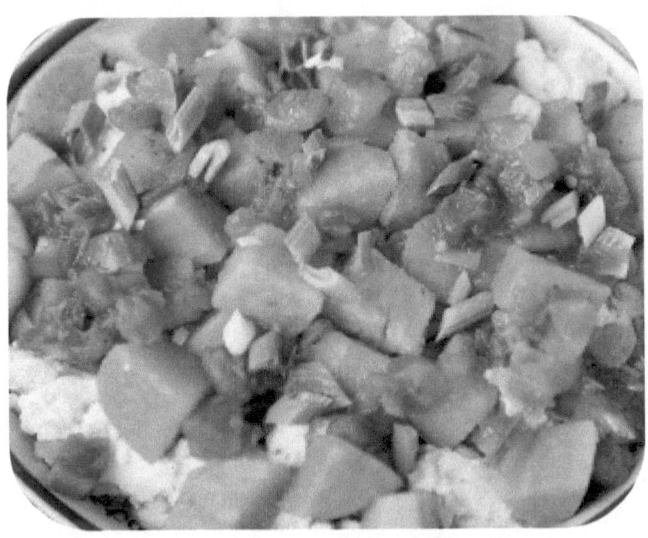

Sweet Potato & Scrambled Eggs

Sweet Potato And Scrambled Eggs

Enjoy this delightful low calorie meal.

Preparation time: 5 minutes

Cooking time: 6 minutes

Servings: 4

Ingredients:

¼ cup of canned full-fat coconut milk

8 eggs

1 large-sized cooked sweet potato, cubed

2 tablespoons of fresh parsley, minced finely

2 tablespoons of ghee or olive oil

1 teaspoon of ground cumin

1 teaspoon of dried oregano

Pepper

Salt

Directions:

1. In a large skillet, heat the ghee over medium heat.

2. In a large bowl, whisk all the ingredients except the potato. Pour this mixture into the skillet and cook until the eggs are almost done. Stir gently.

3. Add the potato cubes, stir to combine and remove from the heat.

Fennel Pudding

Fennel contains fiber and can also help liver detoxification

Preparation time: 10minutes

Cooking time: 50minutes

Servings: 2

Ingredients:

171/2 ounce fennel, chopped coarsely

2 ounce onion, chopped finely

11/2 tbsp butter

2 egg yolks

Salt

Water

Directions:

1. Add the chopped onion, fennel, water and butter to a pan, cover and braise covered until soft and the water evaporates.

2. Puree in a food processor and then set aside to cool.

3. Whisk the egg yolks and some salt together and then add to fennel puree, mixing well.

4. Butter a baking dish and add the mixture.

5. Finally, bake in a preheated oven or at 302° F for 20 to 30 minutes.

Grain- Free Nutty Ginger Cereal

Enjoy this grain-free yummy and satisfying breakfast recipe that can also serve as an alternative to eggs.

Preparation time: 10 minutes

Cooking time: 0 minute

Servings: 6

Ingredients:

1 cup of toasted pecan halves

1/3 cup of toasted unsalted sunflower seeds

1 cup coconut flakes, unsweetened

4 dried dates, diced finely

2 tbsp hemp seeds

¼ tsp dried ginger

¼ tsp dried cinnamon

Directions:

1. Combine the ingredients in a glass jar and store.

2. Enjoy with preferred milk.

Chia Seed Yogurt Meal

Chia is rich in fiber and omega-3 fatty acids and can also help thicken pudding and other custard-like desserts. Enjoy with blackberries and chopped pecans.

Preparation time: 5-10 minutes

Cooking time: 0 minute

Servings: 2

Ingredients:

6 tbsp chia seeds

1/2 tsp ground sumac

1/2 tsp cinnamon

1/4 cup orange juice, squeezed

3/4 cup coconut milk

2 tbsp honey

1/2 tsp vanilla extract

1 cup kefir or plain yogurt

Directions:

1. In a blender, blend the chia seeds, sumac and cinnamon until a coarse-like powder is formed.

2. Next, add the milk, orange juice, yogurt, vanilla and honey.

3. Pulse four to five times in two second increments until the mixture is thick like soup.

4. Refrigerate 1 hour or all night to set well and become as thick as custard.

Pecan-Ginger Cereal

This awesome breakfast will help to soothe hunger and cravings.

Preparation time: 5 minutes

Cooking time: 0 minute

Servings: 6

Ingredients:

1 cup of unsweetened coconut flakes

1 cup of toasted pecan halves

1/3 cup of toasted unsalted sunflower seeds

2 tablespoons of hemp seeds

4 dried dates, finely chopped

¼ teaspoon of dried cinnamon

¼ teaspoon of dried ginger

Directions:

1. Thoroughly combine all the ingredients and place in a glass jar.

2. Serve with milk.

No-Dairy Cornmeal Breakfast

Preparation time: 5 minutes

Cooking time: 5minutes

Servings: 1

Ingredients:

1-1/2 cups unsweetened almond milk

1 cup corn meal (prefer corn grits)

2 cups cold water

Salt

Grapeseed oil

Pure maple syrup (to taste)

Directions:

1. Heat the almond milk in a saucepan.

2. In a bowl, add together corn meal and cold water, stirring well. Now add to the milk in saucepan and stir once more.

 3. Bring to a boil and stir a few times. Lower heat and stir often to prevent it from sticking.

4. Once thick, remove from heat and then season with salt, grapeseed oil and maple syrup.

23

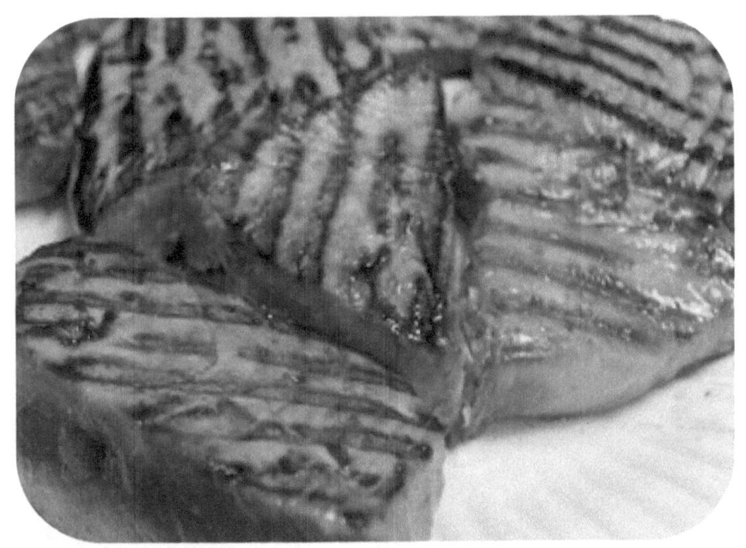

Grilled Tuna Steaks

Packed with protein, this light meal pairs so well with a salad

Preparation time: 4 hours

Cooking time: 10 minutes

Servings: 2

Ingredients:

2 tuna steaks

2 tbsp olive oil or ghee

2 garlic cloves, crushed

Juice and zest of 1 lime

Salt & pepper

1 avocado, sliced

Directions:

1. In a glass bowl, add together all the ingredients except the tuna steaks and avocado.

2. Add the tuna steaks to the bowl and cover thoroughly with the marinade, (use your hands for this).

3. Cover the bowl and refrigerate for 4 hours.

4. Now grill the steaks on medium heat for 5 minutes per side or until cooked to preferred liking

5. Enjoy your steaks with avocado and salad.

Chicken And Grape Salad

Use leftover chicken for this tasty lunch recipe

Preparation time: 5 minutes

Cooking time: 5 minutes

Servings: 4

Ingredients:

1lb leftover cooked chicken

1 cup red or green grapes, halved or left whole

2 hard boiled eggs, sliced

2 stalks celery, sliced

½ cup toasted pecans, chopped

2 large ripe tomatoes, diced

Flesh from 1 avocado, sliced

<u>For Dressing</u>

2 tablespoons olive oil

 2 tablespoons lemon juice

Directions:

1. Combine all the ingredients in a bowl and gently mix.

2. Drizzle with the dressing ingredients, tossing gently.

3. Serve and enjoy!

Succulent Chicken Burgers

Red meat is a no-no when you have fatty liver. However, with this tasty and succulent chicken burger recipe, you wouldn't miss out on anything!

Preparation time: 6 minutes

Cooking time: 10 minutes

Servings: 5

Ingredients:

1 lb ground white meat chicken

2 cups of fresh bread crumbs, divided

1/4 cup of low-fat milk

3 tbsp sweet onion, grated or finely minced

1/4 tsp cayenne pepper

3/4 Kosher salt

Fresh ground black pepper

1 tsp olive oil

Directions:

1. In a mixing bowl, add the chicken, fold in the milk (with a spatula), onion, 1/2 cup bread crumbs, cayenne, salt and pepper.

2. Place the bread crumbs that are left on a plate or cookie sheet.

3. Add olive oil to a large non-stick skillet and heat on medium.

4. Divide chicken meat into portion sizes and shape into patties. (Dampen your hands with water to ease the process). Coat the patty with bread crumbs.

5. Fry the patties about 5 minutes per side until golden.

6. Enjoy with bun of choice or with your favorite accompaniments.

Salmon Orange Salad

This recipe is loaded with protein; it is delicious too!

Preparation time: 5minutes

Cooking time: 5minutes

Servings: 2

Ingredients:

1 cooked salmon fillet, flaked

1 orange, peeled & sliced

1 medium avocado, sliced

1 stalk celery, sliced

½ cup cherry tomatoes, halved

¼ red onion, sliced

¼ cup lime juice

2 tablespoons of olive oil

Salt and pepper, to taste

Directions:

1. Add all salad ingredients to a bowl

2. Top with olive oil and lime juice, mixing well.

Zucchini Caviar

An irresistibly healthy lunch!

Preparation time: 10minutes

Cooking time: 65minutes

Servings: 3

Ingredients:

2 medium carrots, cleaned & chopped into small square-shaped pieces

2 medium zucchinis, cleaned & chopped into small square-shaped pieces

2 big tomatoes

3 pepper, seeded & chopped

2 white onions

Sugar & salt

Olive oil

Directions:

1. Heat the olive oil on high heat. Lower heat; add the carrots and onions and cook 10-15 minutes on medium temperature.

2. Add the chopped zucchini, tomatoes and pepper to pan and cook for 40 to 50 minutes.

3. Season with sugar and salt.

Bulgur Tabbouleh

A great to- go light and fresh lunch recipe that is flavorful as well as healthy.

Preparation time: 15 minutes

Cooking time: 10 minutes

Servings: 2

Ingredients:

1 cup vegetable stock

2/3 cup medium-fine bulgur

1 large tomato, seeded & diced

1 Serrano pepper, seeded & diced

1 bell pepper seeded & diced

1 tsp fresh ginger, grated

1 tsp ancho chili powder

½ cup of chopped fresh cilantro

½ cup of chopped fresh mint

1 tsp olive oil

2 limes (grated zest & juiced)

Directions:

1. Bring the stock to a boil.

2. Place the bulgur in a small sauce pan and pour the stock (broth) over bulgur. Cover to let it soak up liquid for 15 minutes or so.

3. Drain excess broth, fluff with a fork and leave to cool.

4. Toss together the veggies, herbs and spices with lime juice and oil and leave it to marinate for 5 minutes.

5. Add bulgur, and enjoy chilled.

Avocado And Tuna Salad

A Low carb lunch that's quick, easy and delicious!

Preparation time: 15 minutes

Cooking time: 10 minutes

Servings: 1

Ingredients:

1 handful of arugula leaves

½ cup of cherry tomatoes, halved

½ medium avocado, diced

½ Lebanese sliced cucumber

2 tbsp of hemp seeds

5 oz can tuna (with brine), drained & flaked

2 tablespoons olive oil

1 tbsp lime juice or fresh lemon

Directions:

1. Mix all the salad ingredients together.

2. Drizzle with lime juice or lemon and olive oil.

Vegetable Buckwheat Noodle Lunch

A good dish to try when considering liver health.

Preparation time: 5 minutes

Cooking time: 10-15 minutes

Servings: 1

Ingredients:

2 oz or 1¼ cup whole wheat noodle such as organic soba noodles, cooked

¾ cup of broccolini stems, cut along the length

¾ cup bok choy or green cabbage, ribboned

2 tsp toasted sesame oil

2 cups mushroom, vegetable or chicken broth

½ tsp Chinese 5-spice

2 small French breakfast or globe radishes, sliced in coin- shapes

1 small jalapeno (seeded and sliced into coins)

Directions:

1. Cook noodles a minute less than directed on the package, drain and toss with a teaspoon of sesame oil so it doesn't stick.

2. Steam cabbage and broccolini 1 minute.

3. Next, heat a skillet over a medium-high and then add the 1 teaspoon of sesame oil that's left. Add the cabbage and broccolini, sautéing 5 minutes or until just a bit charred. Remove and set aside.

4. Bring the broth to a boil, add the 5 spice and noodles, stirring well; remove.

5. Pour the broth, noodles, and veggies into a bowl. Add chilled radish and jalapeno to top. *Enjoy!*

Spicy Chickpea And Artichoke Sauté

A quick one-pan protein-rich meal that contains fiber and vitamins C and K (thanks to artichoke), which can help with fatty liver and other liver issues.

Preparation time: 5 minutes

Cooking time: 7 minutes

Servings: 4

Ingredients:

1 ½ cup (about 1 can) cooked chickpeas, rinsed

1 ½ cup (about 1 can) artichoke hearts, rinsed

3 tbsp extra virgin olive oil

2 tsp turmeric

½ tsp sea salt

½ tsp cracked black pepper

1 tbsp minced garlic

<u>Optional</u>

1 teaspoon fenugreek seeds

1 teaspoon coriander

1 teaspoon shaved ginger

Directions:

1. Add together artichoke hearts, olive oil, chickpeas and seasonings in a bowl and mix well.

2. Add the ingredients in a preheated hot pan or skillet and shake well so it doesn't stick.

3. Stir once and cook about 6 minutes until the chickpea forms a nicely brown crust.

4. Squeeze over lemon juice. Chill for up to 3 days or enjoy immediately with whole wheat pita bread.

Spinach, Walnut & Apple Lunch

Spinach helps with liver detoxification while apples help to cleanse the liver.

Preparation time: 20 minutes

Cooking time: 5minutes

Servings: 4

Ingredients:

14 ounce spinach leaves, washed & spin-dry

1 heaped tablespoon of cranberries

2 garlic cloves, chopped finely

1 tablespoon olive oil

1.7 ounce walnut kernels

1/5 apple, sliced

Red peppercorns

Salt

Directions:

1. Fry the walnut kernels gently in the pan.

2. Add olive oil, garlic, and apple slices.

3. Add salt and peppercorns to your liking.

Lime Cilantro Cauliflower Lunch

Rich in vitamin C, limes supports liver health. Vitamin C- rich cauliflower is also a great source of vitamin K, niacin and thiamine, which all aids a healthy liver.

Preparation time: 15 minutes

Cooking time: 5minutes

Servings: 4

Ingredients:

1 lime

1 head cauliflower

2 garlic cloves, minced

1 handful cilantro, chopped

Directions:

1. Remove leaves from cauliflower, cut head in half, remove cauliflower from core so only the florets remain.

2. Place half of the cauliflower into the processor and then process to small pieces. Transfer from processor to a pan. Process the other half of the cauliflower; going through the steps once more.

3. Add the minced garlic to the cauliflower in the pan.

4. Now cook for about 5 minutes over medium heat, stirring constantly.

5. Remove from heat when cauliflower is a bit toasted, and the garlic cooked.

6. Toss with cilantro and lime juice.

Cauliflower Fritters

Another healthy cauliflower option to enjoy!

Preparation time: 5 minutes

Cooking time: 35minutes

Servings: 10 fritters

Ingredients:

1 medium head of cauliflower

2 cloves garlic, minced

1/2 tsp chili powder

2 tbsp fresh cilantro, chopped

1/2 tsp fresh ground black pepper

1 1/2 tsp salt

 2 large eggs

1/3 cup flour

4 tbsp cornmeal

2 tablespoons of Coconut oil

5 tbsp nutritional yeast

Directions:

1. Break cauliflower florets down, steam or simmer in water 5 minutes, then drain water, chop (or process) the cauliflower into tiny pieces.

2. Add the cauliflower with the garlic, chili powder, cilantro, salt and pepper, mixing well.

3. Whisk eggs in a separate bowl, and add to cauliflower mixture, together with the flour, corn meal, and nutritional yeast.

4. Add coconut oil to pan, heat up and then add a quarter of the mixture to the pan. Press down the fritter lightly to flatten it.

5. Cook 3 minutes on each side or until golden brown.

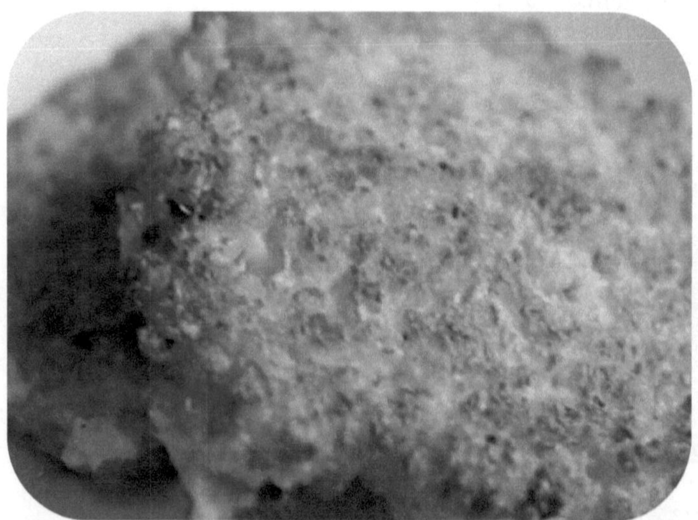

DINNER RECIPES

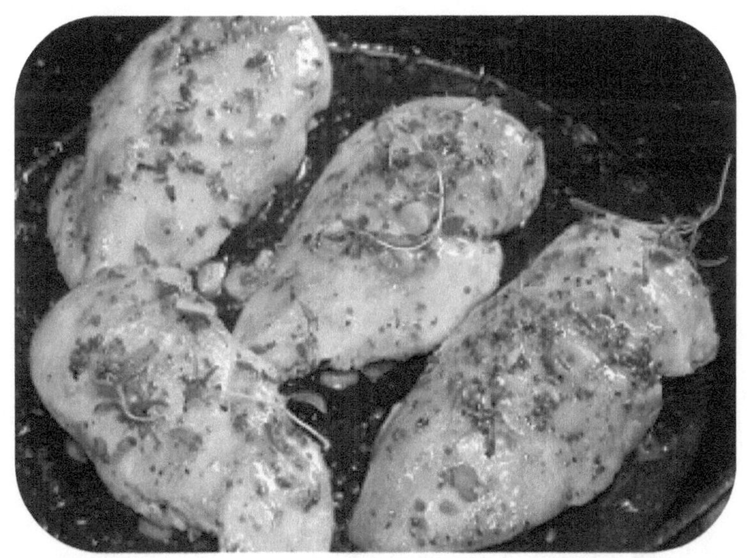

Grainy French Mustard Maple-Glazed Chicken

This special dinner recipe utilizes lean protein and grainy mustard with great flavor.

Preparation time: 5 minutes

Cooking time: 30minutes

Servings: 4

Ingredients:

2 large chicken breasts, (skinless), rinse and pat dry

2 tbsp grainy French mustard

2 tbsp Dijon mustard

1 clove garlic, minced

½ tsp dried thyme

2 tbsp pure maple syrup

Directions:

1. Preheat the oven to 375°F. Butterfly the rinsed and dry chicken breast by cutting in half. However, do not cut all the way through to the other side; but stop about a quarter inch from the other edge of the chicken. Open up the breast (like a book), to make two thinner breasts for quicker cooking, and place in a baking dish.

2. In a small bowl, add together the mustard, thyme, garlic, and maple syrup.

3. Spread about 1½ tablespoons of the mustard mixture equally on top of each chicken breast, (be sure to cover the surface as much as possible in order to form a "crust.")

4. Bake about 25 minutes and then remove. Turn oven to broil, return the chicken to the oven and cook about 4 minutes until the mustard mixtures form a crust and is a little hard.

5. Serve with rice and vegetable.

Herby Mushroom-Flavored Rice Casserole

A stock-rich dish with an earthy mushroom flavor

Preparation time: 5 minutes

Cooking time: 35minutes

Servings: 3

Ingredients:

2 tbsp of unsalted butter

5 chopped green onion (green &white parts)

1 tsp garlic, minced

1 tsp dried oregano

½ tsp cayenne pepper

½ tsp ground black pepper

1 medium bunch fresh parsley, stems off & minced

4 cups chopped mushrooms (oyster, portabello, cremini or trumpet)

2 medium bunches dill, stems off and minced

2 cups of cooked brown rice

1 ½ cup of vegetable stock

Directions:

1. Heat the butter in a large non-stick skillet over medium heat. Add the onion and garlic, stirring about 5 minutes until translucent.

2. Add the pepper, cayenne and oregano, and pepper for an additional minute. Add the dill, parsley and mushrooms, and cook about 10 minutes until the mushrooms are soft,

3. Next, preheat your oven to 350°F.

4. In a 2 ½ quart casserole dish, add the rice and veggie mixture and pour it over the vegetable stock,

5. Do not cover, but bake for 30 minutes.

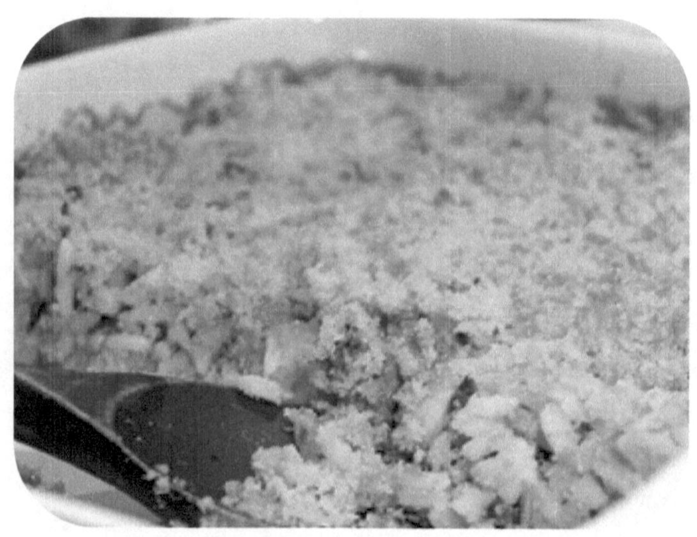

Ground Turkey & Vegetable Stuffed Peppers

Why crave for the traditional beef and rice stuffed pepper, when you can enjoy a healthier dish of Stuffed peppers with ground turkey and vegetables.

Preparation time: 35 minutes

Cooking time: 15minutes

Servings: 4

Ingredients:

4 red bell peppers

1 lb (93%) lean ground turkey

2 tbsp olive oil

1 cup sliced mushrooms

1/2 onion, minced

1 zucchini, chopped

1/2 yellow bell pepper, diced, tops cut off and deseed

1/2 green bell pepper, diced, tops cut off and deseed

1 cup fresh spinach

1 tablespoon tomato paste

1 (14.5 oz) can diced tomatoes, drained

1 tsp Italian seasoning

1/2 tsp garlic powder

Salt and pepper to taste

Directions:

1. Boil a large pot of water. Cook the cut and deseeded peppers (as well as the cut tops) in the boiling water for 5 minutes. Drain the water and set to one side.

2. Preheat oven to 350 degrees F.

3. Cook the turkey in a skillet until well- browned and remove then set aside.

4. Heat the olive oil in the same skillet and then add in the onions, zucchini, peppers, mushrooms and spinach, and let it cook until tender.

5. Place the turkey back to the skillet and add the rest of the ingredients. Stuff the peppers with the mixture

6. Put the peppers inside a casserole dish, replace tops (if you like), and leave it to bake for 15 minutes.

Thai Spicy Seafood Dinner

Enjoy an easy but exotic dish that combines turmeric, red chili, ginger and lime for scrumptious delight.

Preparation time: 10 minutes

Cooking time: 10minutes

Servings: 4

Ingredients:

1½ lb salmon, halibut or red snapper or halibut, washed, patted dry and cut into pieces of 21/2

2 teaspoons of turmeric

½ teaspoon sea salt flakes, divided

2 tbsp ginger, minced

8 shallots, minced

2 tbsp garlic, minced

1 dried red chile, crumbled

2 tablespoons peanut oil

2 limes, halved for squeezing

Directions:

1. In a bowl, toss fish in turmeric and set aside.

2. Grind shallots with half of the sea salt to a paste. Remove to separate bowl.

3. Empty the mortar used in grinding the shallots and grind the remaining salt, ginger and garlic.

4. Add½ tablespoon peanut oil to large skillet and heat on medium. Add the shallot paste and then cook until lightly browned 5 minutes.

5. Add ginger, garlic mixture and chili and then cook 5 more minutes. Add the rest of the oil and then add the fish. Cook for 1 or 2 minutes.

6. Flip and cook 1½ to 2 minutes.

7. Once desired doneness is attained, turn off heat and then squeeze lime juice over it. Enjoy with brown rice.

Grilled Veggie Gratin

Preparation time: 10 minutes

Cooking time: 10minutes

Servings: 4

Ingredients

1/4 cup coconut oil

1/4 tsp dried chili flakes

2 cloves garlic, crushed

1 large eggplant, cut into Slices of 8

2 large zucchini, cut into Slices of 8

3 flat mushrooms, sliced thickly

1 cup tomato pasta sauce

14.8 oz cannellini beans, rinsed &drained

1 cup parmesan cheese, grated

Fresh basil leaves to serve

Directions:

1. Heat your grill plate. In a bowl, add together oil, garlic and chili and brush the veggies with the oil mixture.

2. Oil the grill plate lightly and then cook the veggies until tender. Transfer cooked vegetables to a plate and cover with foil.

3. Meanwhile, add 2/3 cup of the pasta sauce and the beans together, heat in a saucepan until hot and then cover.

4. Preheat grill. Bring out four shallow pasta plate and then place 4 slices of eggplant, 1/4 zucchini, mushrooms & bean mixture in them. Top with the eggplant slices that are left and remaining pasta sauce. Sprinkle with cheese.

5. Place under your preheated grill 3 minutes. Remove once cheese is melted and lightly browned. Top with Basil.

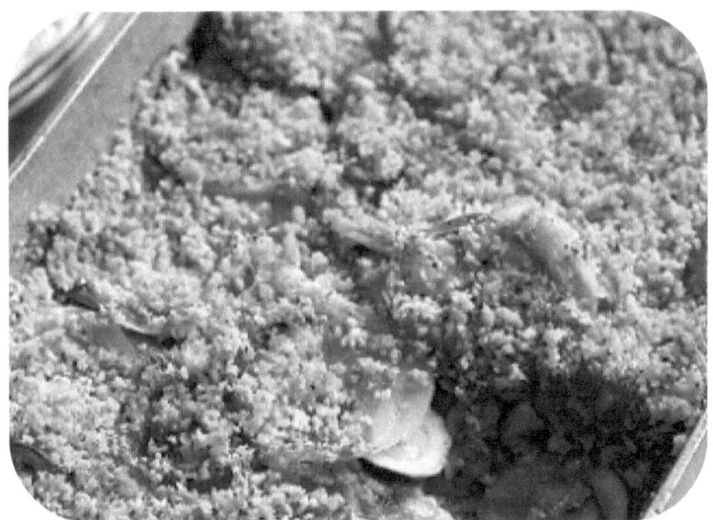

Lemon Poached Chicken

As a natural cleanser, Lemon cleans your body of toxins; chicken is also loaded with lean protein, which is good for your liver.

Preparation time: 10minutes

Cooking time: 30 minutes

Servings: 3

Ingredients

3 lb chicken breast

4 garlic cloves, cracked but whole

4 quarts chicken stock

½ onion yellow, diced largely

1 lemon, halved

4 thyme sprigs

1 tsp black peppercorns

Directions:

1. In a small pot, add all the ingredients and bring to a simmer. Cook 25-30 minutes, remove the chicken from stock and set aside.

2. Serve immediately or refrigerate for later.

3. Strain, cool, and refrigerate stock for up to 1 week for future use.

Softly Grilled Baby Octopus

Preparation time: 6 hours

Cooking time: 10minutes

Servings: 4

Ingredients

2lb baby octopus, cleaned& trimmed

½ cup olive oil

¼ cup lime juice or lemon

1 tsp freshly grated lemon or lime zest

2 cloves garlic, crushed

½ tsp salt

Directions:

1. Add 5 cups of water to a large pot and bring to a boil. Turn off the heat and add the octopuses. Let it sit1minute, drain and rinse under cold water.

2. Combine the rest of the ingredients together in a bowl, preferably glass. Add the octopuses, covering them all in. Cover the bowl and refrigerate about 6 hours.

3. Enjoy with a salad.

Whole-Wheat Spaghetti With Salmon, Lemon And Basil

A healthy meal with protein and omega-3 rich salmon.

Preparation time: 10 minutes

Cooking time: 10 minutes

Servings: 4

Ingredients:

1/2 lb whole grain or whole wheat spaghetti

2 tbsp extra-virgin olive oil

1 clove garlic, minced

1/2 tsp salt, + more for seasoning

1/2 tsp freshly ground black pepper, + more for seasoning

1 tbsp olive oil

4 (4-oz) pieces wild caught, Alaskan salmon

1/4 cup fresh basil leaves, chopped

3 tbsp capers

1 lemon, zested

2 tbsp lemon juice

2 cups fresh baby spinach leaves

Directions:

1. Cook pasta 8-10 minutes until al dente; drain and toss in a large bowl along with the extra-virgin olive oil, garlic, salt & pepper. Set aside.

2. In a medium skillet over medium-high temperature, warm the olive oil.

3. Now season the salmon with some salt and pepper and add to the skillet and cook until about 2 minutes per side or to your desire likeness. Remove fish from pan.

4. Add the capers, basil, lemon juice and lemon zest to the spaghetti mixture and toss well to combine.

5. Place 1/2 cup of spinach each in 4 bowls. Top with 1/4 pasta and then top with salmon. Enjoy!

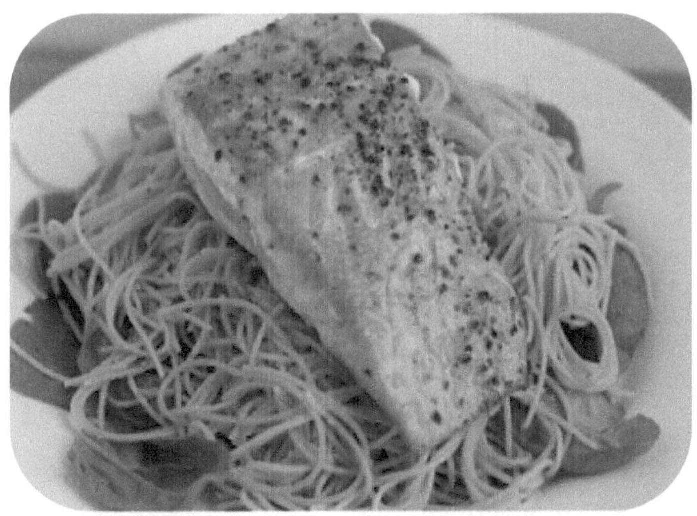

Leftover Turkey With Squash Soup

A healthy soup with butternut squash chunks to enjoy with friends and family

Preparation time: 14 minutes

Cooking time: 40 minutes

Servings: 4

Ingredients:

2 leeks, trimmed, chopped &rinsed

2 tsp canola oil

3 cloves garlic, minced

1 red bell pepper, chopped

4 cups reduced-sodium chicken broth

1 1/2 lb butternut squash, peeled, seeded and cut into cubes of1-inch

2 teaspoons dried thyme or 2 tbsp minced fresh thyme

1 1/2 tsp ground cumin

4 cups leftover turkey, shredded

2 cups frozen corn kernels

2 tbsp fresh lime juice

1/2 teaspoon red pepper, crushed

1/4 tsp salt

Freshly ground pepper, to taste

Directions:

1. In a Dutch oven, heat oil over medium-high heat. Add the leeks and bell pepper; cook and stir continuously, 3 to 4 minutes until soften.

2. Add garlic, cook and stir another minute. Add the squash, broth, thyme & cumin; cover and let it boil. Set heat to medium-low and cook about 10 minutes until tender.

3. Add the turkey and corn; let it simmer and cook 2 to 3 minutes until just heated through.

4. Add the lime juice and crushed red pepper. Add salt and pepper to taste. *Enjoy!*

Chicken Dumpling Soup

Enjoy this delicious dinner meal that includes garlic, a great source of prebiotic soluble fiber to help liver patients.

Preparation time: 30minutes

Cooking time: 2 hours 30 minutes

Servings: 6

Ingredients:

2 teaspoons of avocado oil

2lbs chicken breast, diced largely

2 cups onion, diced

1 cup carrot, diced

1 cup celery, diced

3teaspoons of garlic, minced

1 leek bottom, medium diced

2tsp black pepper, fresh cracked

2tbsp thyme chopped

1tsp rosemary, minced

3qts of water

1 bay leaf

2 tablespoons of cornstarch + 2tbsp water

24 tablespoons of gluten-Free biscuit dough

Directions:

1. Heat avocado oil over medium high heat and then add the chicken. Cook until browned.

2. Stir in the veggies and cook until the onions are tender. Add your spices and aromatics and cook until fragrant.

3. Add water. Cover and simmer 2hrs. Whisk in the cornstarch mixture and simmer, stirring continuously.

4. Add the biscuit dough to the soup. Cover and let cook 15 - 20 minutes. Enjoy!

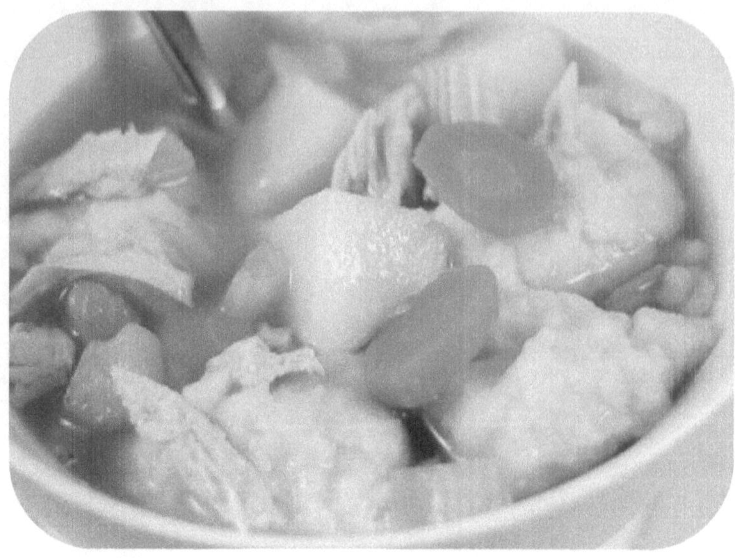

SALAD RECIPES

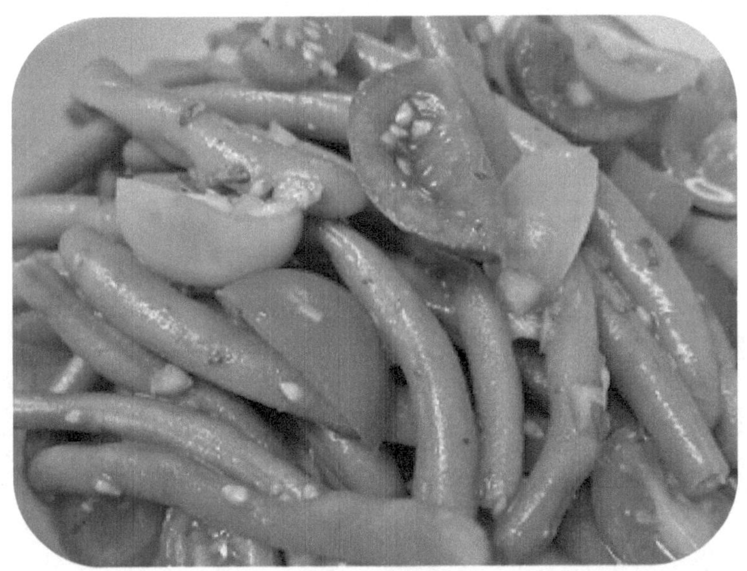

Anti-Fatty Liver Potato Salad

Boost your health (and your liver, of course) with this great salad recipe.

Preparation time: 3 minutes

Cooking time: 10-15 minutes

Servings: 6-8

Ingredients:

4 large potatoes, cubed about an inch

1/2 cup lemon juice

2 tsp turmeric or mustard powder

1/2 tsp of cumin seeds (optional)

1 1/2 tsp sea salt

1 red small onion, chopped finely

2 cloves garlic, minced

1/2 cup of extra virgin olive oil

2 tbsp of fresh parsley, chopped

Directions:

1. Steam the potatoes for about 15 minutes until fork tender.

2. Combine the lemon juice, turmeric or mustard powder, cumin seeds (if using) and lastly salt.

3. Add the steamed potatoes to a bowl, pour over the lemon juice mixture, add the garlic and onions and stir carefully to cover the potatoes. Cover and remove to cool in a refrigerator.

4. Once cool, pour over olive oil, add the parsley and stir well.

5. Enjoy chilled or at room temperature.

Green Bean& Cherry Tomato Salad

Preparation time: 5 minutes

Cooking time: 2 minutes

Servings: 4

Ingredients:

4 handfuls green beans, steamed lightly

1 cup cherry tomatoes, halved

¼ red onion, sliced

1 large carrot, grated coarsely

2 handfuls arugula leaves, chopped roughly

¼ cup pine nuts, toasted

3 tablespoons olive oil

¼ cup red wine vinegar

Directions:

1. Add together all the ingredients in a serving bowl and gently toss.

2. Serve with chicken or seafood of choice.

Hungarian Cucumber Salad

Enjoy with any protein of choice

Preparation time: 5minutes

Cooking time: 2 hours

Servings: 8

Ingredients:

2 English cucumbers, peeled & thinly sliced

1/2 onion, cut into paper-thin slices

2 tbsp seasoned Salt

1/2 cup white vinegar

1/4 cup water

2 tsp sugar

1 tsp sweet Hungarian paprika

1 tbsp sour cream (optional)

Pinch of dill, dried or fresh (optional)

Directions:

1. Place the peeled and sliced cucumbers on a large baking sheet and sprinkle with salt, until thoroughly salted. Let it rest 30 minutes.

2. Place the sliced onions in a bowl. Rinse the cucumber slices in a colander and squeeze out excess water.

3. Now add the now limp but crisp cucumbers to the onions. Add the water, vinegar, sugar, and paprika to it. Leave the cucumber and onions to marinate for 1 ½-2 hours in the refrigerator.

4. Remove from the fridge, and add the dill (if using), and serve. To add the sour cream (if using), let the onion and cucumber marinate, pour off some of liquid and then mix in the sour cream.

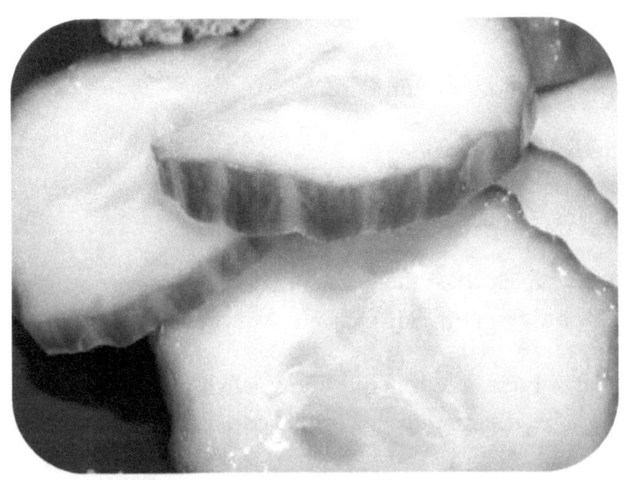

Strawberry Spinach Salad

A healthy dish that contains spinach to help liver detoxification process.

Preparation time: 5minutes

Cooking time: 15minutes

Servings: 8

Ingredients:

1 cup of roasted pecans

12 oz baby spinach & mixed field greens mix

16 oz strawberries, sliced or quartered

1/2 cup of olive oil

1/4 cup of balsamic vinaigrette

4 tsp Dijon mustard

Balsamic Vinaigrette Dressing:

1/2 cup olive oil

4 teaspoons Dijon mustard

1/4 cup balsamic vinaigrette

Directions:

1. In a dry skillet, toast the pecans over medium-low heat, about 10 to 15 minutes until fragrant. Stir frequently to prevent scorching.

2. In a large bowl, add together the spinach mix, pecans and strawberries. Add the salad dressing tossing until coated evenly.

3. Combine all the ingredients for the dressing. Add salt to taste, if you like.

Super Greens Mix
Preparation time: 15minutes

Cooking time: minutes

Servings: 1

Ingredients:

1/4 bag of baby leaf spinach, rinsed & dried

1/4 bag watercress, rinsed & dried

Handful basil leaves

1tablespoon of EVOI (extra virgin olive oil)

Handful parsley leaves

Squeeze of lemon juice

Directions:

1. In a food processor, process all the ingredients or chop or cut the herbs finely and add the oil and stir well.

Greek Salad

Please your palate with this colorful Greek salad.

Preparation time: 45minutes

Cooking time: minutes

Servings: 6

Ingredients:

Salad:

1 English cucumber, unpeeled, seeded & sliced to 1/4-inch thickness

1 yellow bell pepper, seeded and diced largely

1 orange bell pepper, seeded and diced largely

1 pint grape tomatoes, halved

1/2 red onion, sliced in half-rounds

1/2 cup black or Kalamata olives, pitted

4 oz feta cheese (optional)

Vinaigrette:

2 cloves garlic, minced

1 teaspoon oregano, dried

1/2 tsp Dijon mustard

1/4 cup red wine vinegar

1 tsp kosher salt

1/2 tsp freshly ground black pepper

1/2 cup olive oil

Directions:

1. In a large bowl, place the tomatoes, cucumber, red onion and pepper.

2. In a separate bowl, combine the garlic, mustard, oregano, vinegar, salt and pepper, whisking well. Still whisking, gently add the olive oil.

3. Pour the vinaigrette over the veggies, add the feta (if using) and olives, tossing lightly.

4. Let it stay for 30 minutes to blend the flavors. Serve at room temperature.

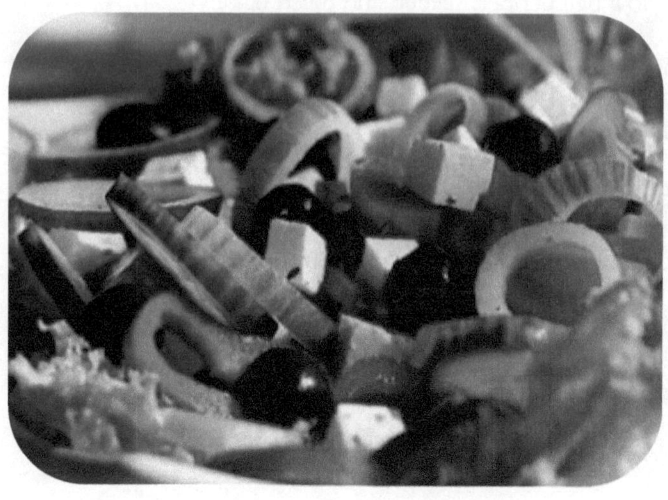

Pickled Cucumber Salad

Enjoy this salad dish of vitamin and fiber rich cucumbers and cucumbers; and Quercetin-rich red onions that are good for your liver.

Preparation time: 30minutes

Cooking time: minutes

Servings: 1

Ingredients:

3 cups cucumbers peeled, seeded, sliced

¼ cup red onion, sliced thinly

½ cup red bell pepper, chopped

Dressing:

2 tablespoons coconut aminos

1 tablespoon rice vinegar

1 tbsp toasted sesame oil

2 tsp honey

2 tbsp cilantro or green onion, sliced

1 tablespoon sesame seeds

Preparation time: 30 minutes

Directions:

1. To a large bowl, place the cucumbers, red bell pepper and red onion.

2. Add the soy sauce, sesame oil, rice vinegar, honey, sesame seeds and cilantro to a small bowl, whisking well. Season with salt and pepper as desired.

3. Pour dressing over the vegetables and toss well to coat.

4. Serve immediately or refrigerate for up to 8 hours.

Rubbed Kale Salad With Other Ingredients

Reduce the bitterness of kale by adding other ingredients in this recipe. It also softens its texture. Enjoy!

Preparation time: 20minutes

Cooking time: minutes

Servings: 4

Ingredients:

1 large bunch kale (stalk removed and sliced round)

Juice of 1lemon

1/4 extra-virgin olive oil, plus extra for drizzling

2 teaspoons honey

Kosher salt

Freshly ground black pepper

1 cup dried cranberries

2 heaping tbsp toasted pepitas/pumpkin seeds

Directions:

1. Add the kale, some kosher salt and half lemon juice to a mixing bowl.

2. Use your fingertips to rub the kale for 5 minutes. Once the leaves are tender, drizzle olive oil and rub 1 more minute.

3. In a small bowl, add the rest of the lemon juice, honey and freshly ground black pepper, whisking well. Whisk in 1/4 cup of the oil until a dressing forms. Now add salt to taste.

4. Pour some dressing over the kale to coat, and add the cranberries and pepitas. Toss well and serve.

Colorful Fruit Salad

Preparation time: 20minutes

Cooking time: minutes

Servings: 2-6

Ingredients:

Strawberries, sliced into 1-inch chunks

Blueberries

Bananas, sliced into 1-inch chunks

Grapes

Fresh Pineapple, sliced into 1-inch chunks

Watermelon, cut into 1-inch chunks

Cantaloupe, cut into 1-inch chunks

1-2 Fresh Lemons or Limes

Optional:

Almonds

Pecans

 Walnuts

Directions:

1. Add together the prepared fruit with grapes and blueberries in a large serving bowl.

2. Squeeze juice of lemons or limes over colorful fruit, mixing gently.

3. Add nuts, if using. Cover and chill.

Multi Bean Salad

Preparation time: 15 minutes

Cooking time: minutes

Servings: 4

Ingredients:

1 cup black beans

1 cup pinto beans

1 cup Garbanzo beans

1 cup of red kidney beans

1 onion, chopped

1 bunch cilantro, chopped

½ cup seasoned rice vinegar

 Salt & Pepper

Directions:

1. Rinse all the beans thoroughly, strain them and place in a bowl.

2. To the beans; add the chopped onion and stir in the rice vinegar.

3. Sprinkle it with salt and pepper.

4. If desired, add chopped green beans, cooked brown rice or olives to enhance the taste.

SOUPS

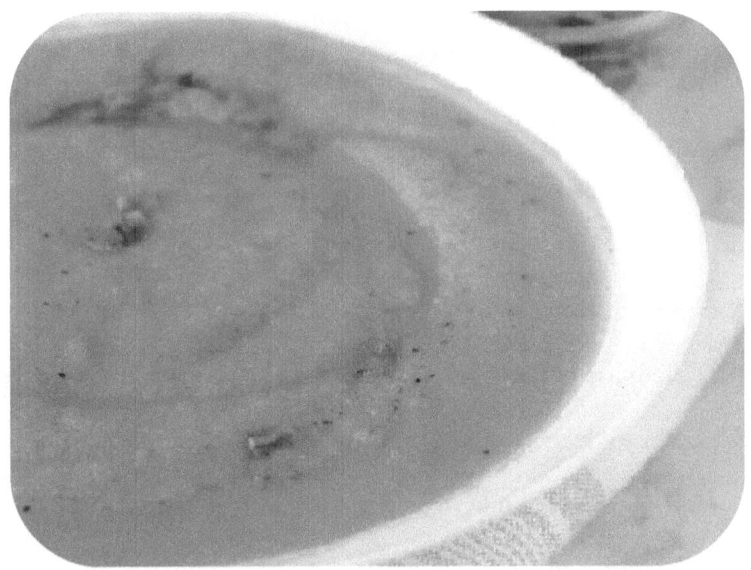

Turkey With Squash Soup

A healthy soup with chunks of nutrient-rich butternut squash

Preparation time: 15 minutes

Cooking time: 40minutes

Servings: 6

Ingredients:

2 tsp canola oil

2 leeks, (trim it, chop it & rinse)

3 cloves garlic, minced

1 red bell pepper, (chop it)

4 cups of chicken broth (reduced-sodium)

1 1/2 lb butternut squash, (peel it, remove seed & cut into cubes of1-inch

2 tbsp fresh thyme, (minced) or 2 tsp of dried thyme

1 1/2 tsp ground cumin

4 cups leftover turkey, shredded

2 cups frozen corn kernels

2 tbsp of fresh lime juice

1/2 tsp red pepper, crushed

1/4 tsp salt

Freshly ground pepper, to taste

Directions:

1. In a Dutch oven, heat oil in over medium-high heat. Add the bell pepper and leeks, cooking and stirring 3 to 4 minutes, until soften.

2. Add the garlic and let it cook while stirring another minute. Stir in broth, cumin, thyme and squash, cover and bring to a boil.

3. Lower heat to medium-low and cook about 10 minutes until tender.

4. Add the turkey and corn; let it simmer and cook 2 to 3 minutes until just heated through.

5. Finally, add lime juice and crushed red pepper. Add salt and pepper to taste. *Enjoy!*

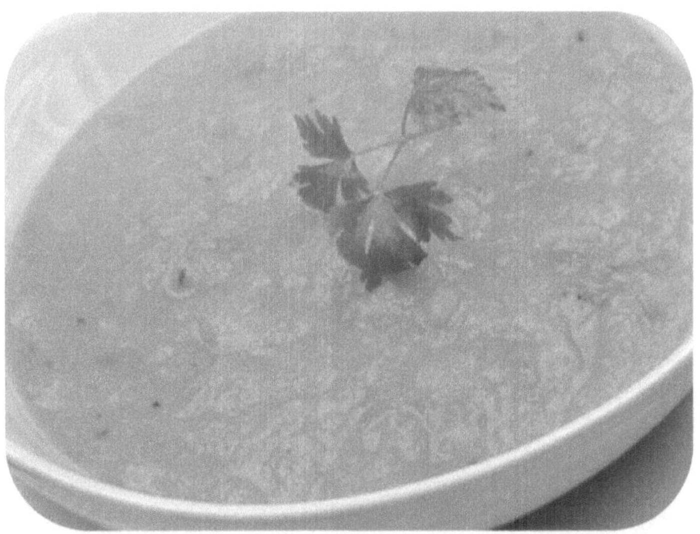

Pear & Red Pepper Soup

Unripe pears are the best. Pick hard pears and leave on your counter to ripen. They have a slightly, sweet flavor that's just right for both sweet and savory dishes.

Preparation time: 25 minutes

Cooking time: 40minutes

Servings: 7

Ingredients:

2 tbsp butter

2 tsp olive oil

2 carrots, sliced

3 large red bell peppers, sliced

2 Anjou pears, (peel & slice it)

2 shallots, cut

1/2 teaspoon dried crushed red pepper

1 (32-oz.) container chicken broth, fat-free

1/4 tsp salt

1/2 tsp ground black pepper

Dash ground red pepper

For Garnishing:

Fresh pears, thinly sliced

Plain yogurt

Fresh chives, chopped

Directions:

1. Add oil to a Dutch oven and melt butter over medium heat; add the bell pepper, carrots, shallots and pears and sauté for about 10 minutes.

2. Once tender, add the chicken broth, stir and then add the peppers, salt and ground red pepper. Bring to a boil; cover, set heat to low, and simmer about 30 minutes. Set aside to cool for 20 minutes.

3. In a food processor, process soup, in batches, until smooth, ensuring to scrape down sides.

4. Place back to Dutch oven, and let it warm up until ready to serve. Garnish, as desired.

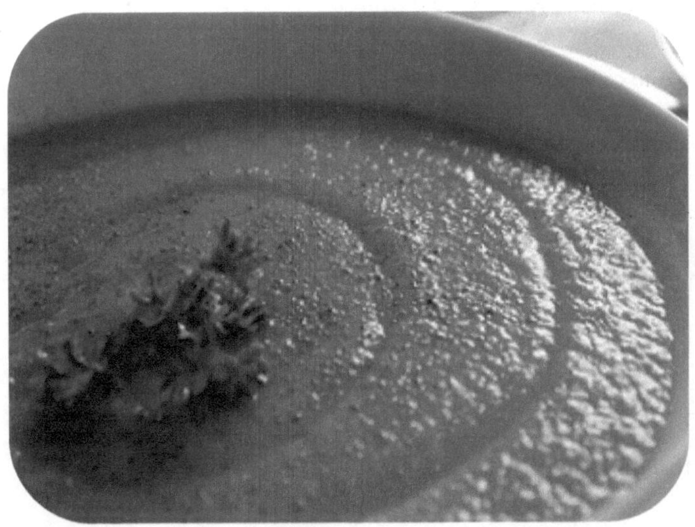

Beet Detox Soup

Delicious and nutritious pink colored beet soup to your delight.

Preparation time: 25 minutes

Cooking time: 45minutes

Servings: 2

Ingredients:

3 medium beet roots

2 carrots, diced finely

1 onion, diced finely

2 garlic cloves, crushed

1 small leek, diced finely

1 teaspoon coconut oil

¼ tsp sea salt

2 cups of warm vegetable broth

For Garnishing:

1 tbsp chia, sunflower

1tbsp pumpkin seeds

1 teaspoon coconut milk

Directions:

1. Place the beet roots in a pot, pour in water to cover, bring to boil and simmer until tender for 30 minutes. Drain and cool.

2. In a cast iron skillet, heat the coconut oil, add in the onions, carrot, leek and garlic and cook over low heat for 5-7 minutes. Remove onto a plate.

3. Now peel the beet roots and cut them into cubes, place in the blender, along with the cooked veggie and the warm vegetable broth.

4. Process until smooth. Add salt garnish with mixed seeds and serve.

Broccoli Soup

A detox soup that's good for your liver.

Preparation time: 15 minutes

Cooking time: 15minutes

Servings: 2

Ingredients:

2 cups broccoli florets

1 onion, finely diced

2 celery stalks, finely diced

2 garlic cloves, crushed

1 cup kale or spinach

1 carrot, peeled &finely chopped

1 parsnip, peeled & finely chopped

2 cups vegetable broth, low sodium or filtered water

½ tsp sea salt

½ lemon, juice only

1 tbsp chia seeds

1 tsp coconut oil

Toasted mixed seeds and nuts

1 tsp coconut milk, to garnish

Directions:

1. Add the coconut oil to a soup pot and heat. Once hot, add the onion, garlic, parsnip, celery, carrot, broccoli and sticks. Lower heat and cook 5 minutes, stirring often.

2. Add the broth or filtered water, bring to a boil, then cover pot and let simmer for 5 to 7 minutes, until the veggies are tender.

3. Add the greens, stir and then remove contents to blender. Now add the chia seeds and lemon, and blend until smooth.

4. Top soup with toasted seeds.

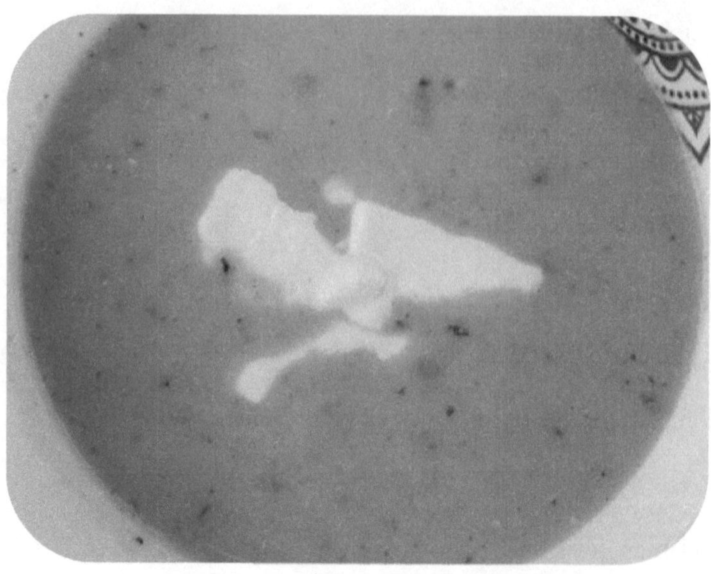

Sweet-Potato Soup

A vitamin A and fiber-packed detox soup for fatty liver.

Preparation time: 5 minutes

Cooking time: 25minutes

Servings: 6

Ingredients:

½ cup of cooked red lentils

1 sweet potato, peeled& cubed

3 carrots, peeled & chopped roughly

1 parsnip, peeled & chopped roughly

1 onion, peeled & quartered

3 garlic cloves, crushed

1 tsp turmeric powder

1 teaspoon of cumin powder

Pinch of chili powder

¼ tsp sea salt

2 cups of warm low sodium vegetable broth

½ inch piece of ginger, peeled & grated

1 teaspoon coconut oil

Fresh parsley, 1 tsp coconut milk, to garnish

Directions:

1. Heat the oven at 329°F.

2. Add the sweet potato, parsnip, carrots, garlic and onion to a lined baking sheet and season with salt, turmeric, chili & cumin. Add the coconut oil, tossing well.

3. Roast 20 minutes then remove to a blender.

4. Add warm vegetable broth, ginger, and red lentils into the blender and blend until smooth.

5. Garnish with fresh parsley and serve warm.

Green Bean Soup
A healthy casserole dish to try

Preparation time: 15 minutes

Cooking time: 45minutes

Servings: 2

Ingredients:

2 tablespoons of butter

½ cup onion, diced

2 cloves garlic, minced

1 cup mushrooms, thinly sliced & diced

3 tablespoons of white whole wheat flour

1½ cups skim milk

½ tsp salt

1 | 2 cups plain Greek yogurt

¾ teaspoon onion powder

¾ teaspoon garlic powder

Black pepper, to taste

24 oz frozen green beans

¼ cup Panko breadcrumbs

¼ cup Parmesan cheese, grated (optional)

Directions:

1. Preheat oven to 350 degrees.

2. Melt butter in a saucepan and add the onion, garlic, mushrooms, sautéing about 5 minutes until soft.

3. Add flour, stir well and cook 2 minutes to remove the raw taste of the flour.

4. Add milk slowly; stirring continuously so it doesn't clump.

5. Add yogurt, onion, salt, garlic black pepper. Lower heat and let it simmer for 5 to 10 minutes until it thickens.

6. Add the green beans to the sauce and stir well to combine.

Vegetable Barley Soup

A dish that's high in fiber, vitamins, minerals and antioxidants for your heart and liver.

Preparation time: 15 minutes

Cooking time: 1 hour 10 minutes

Servings: 6

Ingredients:

2 tbsp olive oil

2 cups of yellow onion diced

½ cup celery, diced

½ cup carrot, diced

3 each garlic cloves, thinly sliced

2 each bay leaf

1 cup tomato diced

½ cup zucchini, diced

1 cup kale, diced

6 cups stock

1 cup cooked barley

1 tbsp parsley fresh

¼ tsp oregano dried

Directions:

1. Sauté oil, onion, garlic, celery, carrots and bay leaf in a medium stock pot.

2. Once translucent, add zucchini, kale and tomato. Cook for 3 minutes, and then add stock and oregano.

3. Simmer 30 minutes and then add barley and fresh parsley. Cook another15 minutes. Serve and enjoy!

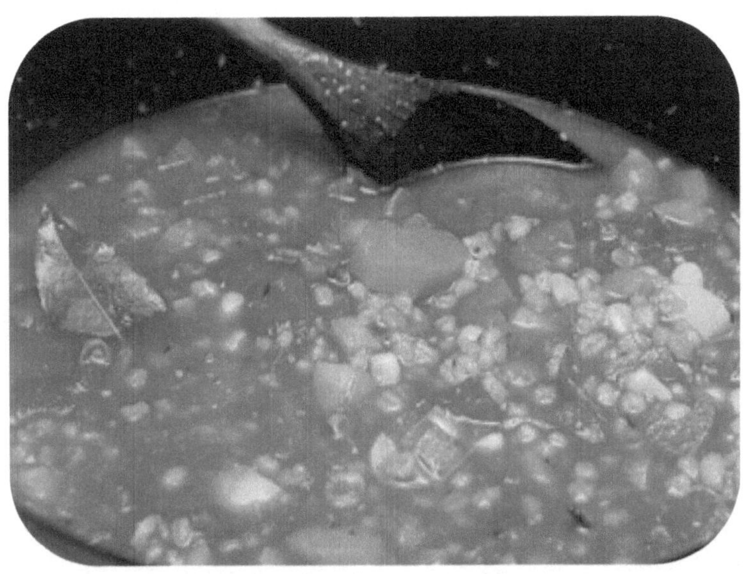

Highly-Spiced Tomato Basil Soup

A healthy dish with liver health benefits

Preparation time: 15 minutes

Cooking time: 30 minutes

Servings: 6

Ingredients:

2 tbsp olive oil

¼ cup oil

¼ cup celery, diced small

1 cup yellow onion, diced

¼ cup carrots, small diced

10 garlic cloves, minced

1 tbsp crushed red pepper

2 bay leaf

8 cups tomato, diced

4 cups vegetable broth

2 tbsp fresh basil

2 tsp black pepper cracked

Directions:

1. Add oil to pot, heat and then add the onion and the celery, along with the garlic, carrots, red pepper and barley, sautéing until the onions are translucent.

 2. Add broth, tomatoes and pepper. Let it simmer and lessen by half.

3. Now add basil and blend or process until smooth.

4. Top with more basil, if you like. *Enjoy!*

Lentil And Kale Soup

Contains the superfood– kale.

Preparation time: 5 minutes

Cooking time: 20 minutes

Servings: 4-6

Ingredients:

1 bunch of kale, stemmed and coarsely chopped

8 cups of vegetable stock

1½ cups of red lentils, rinsed

1 tablespoon of chopped parsley

2 onions, chopped

2 carrots, chopped

1 garlic clove

Zest of ½ a lemon

¼ teaspoon of red pepper flakes, optional

Directions:

1. Put the kale, lentils, stock, garlic, onions and carrots in a large pot. Allow to boil and cook for about 15-20 minutes until the lentils are soft.

2. Add the pepper flakes, lemon zest and parsley. Stir and serve.

Carrot Soup

Preparation time: 20minutes

Cooking time: 20 minutes

Servings: 1

Ingredients:

1 ounce fresh ginger, peeled & chopped finely

7 ounce carrots, washed, peeled &sliced thinly

2 tbsp butter

1/2 tbsp sugar

11|4 cup vegetable stock

1|4 cup Coconut milk

Salt and pepper to taste

Directions:

1. Cook the ginger and carrots in butter and sprinkle over with sugar.

2. Add the stock and coconut milk and bring to boil.

3. Simmer over medium heat for about 20 minutes, and then blend for a smooth consistency.

4. Season with salt and pepper.

Lemon Rice Soup

A flavorful soup you'll love.

Preparation time: 15 minutes

Cooking time: 35 minutes

Servings: 4-8

Ingredients:

1-2 lbs. chicken (thighs legs, breasts or whole chicken)

1 10oz. bag spinach, fresh or frozen

1 large onion yellow, red or white, finely chopped

6-8 garlic cloves, finely chopped

1 jar of roasted red peppers

1 cup orzo, brown rice or couscous

3 tablespoons of lemon juice

5-6 cups water

Directions:

1. Add water, chicken, garlic and onions to a large pot and bring to boil.

2. Remove chicken, cool broth, skim off any fat, and take out skin from chicken. Take out chicken meat from bones, chop meat into bite size pieces and return to broth.

3. Now add bag of spinach, orzo, couscous or rice, along with lemon juice and red peppers. Bring to a boil once more, and then let it simmer until cooked.

4. Freeze if desired, add bouillon, if desired

Tortellini Soup

Enjoy this great tomato based soup, very brothy, with fresh veggies and tortellini to relish for again and again.

Preparation time: 8 minutes

Cooking time: 25 minutes

Servings: 4-6

Ingredients:

2 tbsp of olive oil

1-2 medium-sized carrots, peeled & diced

2 small zucchini, diced

1 or 2 celery stalks, cut thinly

1 potato, peeled & diced

4 scallions

2 quarts low sodium chicken stock

1 large can crushed tomatoes

½ teaspoon salt

0-12oz fresh or frozen tortellini (cheese or meat filled)

Black pepper, to taste

Directions:

1. In a large saucepan, heat the olive oil on medium heat. Add the carrots, zucchini, potato, celery, and scallions. Sauté and stir10 minutes until softened.

2. Add the stock, the tomatoes, and then salt. Set heat to high and bring mixture to a boil.

3. Add the tortellini, bring back the soup to a low boil and then cook 2 minutes. Lower heat and simmer another 5 to 6 minutes.

4. During the last 1-2 minutes, add the pepper, stirring gently.

Simple Basic Soup

Preparation time: 10 minutes

Cooking time: 20 minutes

Servings: 2-3

Ingredients:

1tbsp coconut oil

1/2 red onion, chopped roughly

1 garlic clove, crushed

1 large carrot, peeled & chopped

1 large sweet potato, chopped

1 heaped teaspoon fresh root ginger, grated

1/4teaspoon turmeric

2tsp salt vegetable bouillon powder

75ml coconut milk

1/2 red pepper, diced

Directions:

1. Heat the oil in a large pan and gently sauté the onion and garlic for a few minutes until softened.

2. Now add the carrot and the sweet potato, along with the turmeric, bouillon powder and the ginger. Add boiling water to cover and let it boil. Close lid and simmer 15 minutes.

3. Once veggie softens, add the coconut milk and red pepper, and then blend well until smoothened and thick.

DESSERTS

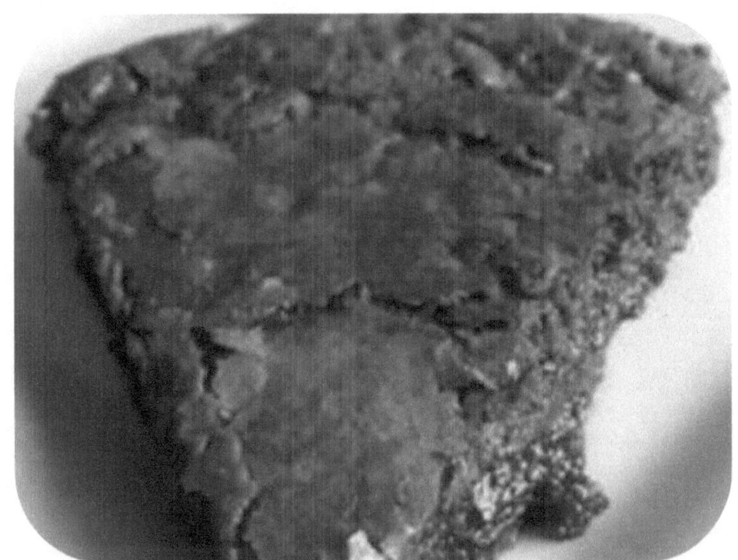

Mini – Banana Pudding

Preparation time: 10 minutes

Cooking time: 20minutes

Servings: 6

Ingredients:

10 whole almonds

2 tbsp cornstarch

Dash of salt, kosher or sea salt

3 tbsp coconut palm sugar

1 egg yolk, slightly beaten

3/4 cup milk, 1 or 2% is recommended

1/2 tsp vanilla

2 bananas, sliced thinly

6 (4 oz) dessert dishes

Directions:

1. Preheat your oven to 325°F. Roast the almonds for 12 minutes and cool. Once cooled, mince the almonds.

2. While you wait, make the pudding by combining cornstarch, sugar and salt. Add the egg yolk, stir in milk gradually and keep stirring until well combined. Lower heat to medium and cook while stirring continuously. Keep cooking until it forms a pudding-like consistency.

3. Remove from heat, add the vanilla and stir well. Alternate the pudding with bananas. Sprinkle the minced almonds over the pudding. *Enjoy!*

Watermelon & Lime Popsicles

A welcome treat on a hot day

Preparation time: 5 minutes

Cooking time: minutes

Servings: 6 popsicles

Ingredients:

1 lb watermelon flesh

2 tablespoons of lime juice

Optional: honey, maple syrup, or stevia, to taste

Directions:

1. Blend ingredients until smooth.

2. Strain through a sieve or leave as it is.

3. Pour mixture into Popsicle molds and freeze until solid.

No-Dairy Peppermint Mousse

Preparation time: 5minutes

Cooking time: 0minutes

Servings: 3

Ingredients:

2 ripe avocados, flesh only

1/3 cup of coconut oil, melted

¼ cup cocoa powder or cacao

1 tsp vanilla essence

1-2 tsp peppermint essence

Honey, maple syrup or liquid stevia, for sweetening according to taste

Directions:

1. Transfer all the ingredients to a blender and blend thoroughly until smooth

2. If too thick, add some water.

Frozen Strawberry Yogurt

Strawberries and low fat yogurts deliver great liver health benefits

Preparation time: 5minutes

Cooking time: 0minutes

Servings: 4

Ingredients:

4 cups organic strawberries

3 tbsp agave nectar

½ cup Greek yogurt

1 tablespoon lemon juice

Directions:

1. Place all the ingredients in a blender or food processor and blend until it is smooth and creamy.

2. Serve immediately or freeze for later.

Super Chocolate Fudge Pie

Get everyone raving about this delicious pie. People will even doubt its tofu content!

Preparation time: 5minutes

Cooking time: 0minutes

Servings: 8-10 slices

Ingredients:

12.3 oz silken or firm tofu

1 1/2 teaspoon of cocoa powder

1 teaspoon of pure vanilla extract

2 tablespoon, milk of choice

1/8 teaspoon of salt

8-10 oz chocolate chips (about 1 1/2 cups)

2-3 teaspoons sweetener of choice

Extracts, liqueurs flavorings, optional

Directions:

1. Melt the chocolate carefully.

2. Remove to a food processor and blend well until smooth. If desired, pour into a pie crust.

3. Place in a refrigerator until chilled. The more it sits, the firmer it gets.

Healthy Avocado Mango Ice Cream

Enjoy this beautiful, icy smoothie. It's healthy too!

Preparation time: 5minutes

Cooking time: 0minutes

Servings: 1

Ingredients:

1 frozen banana

1/2 frozen avocado

1/2 cup frozen mango

1/2 cup spinach or any greens

1 tablespoon Further Food Collagen

Directions:

1. Blend all the ingredients until smooth.

Baked Stone Fruits

A brilliantly healthy dessert with good source of natural sugars; however, it's not ideal for FODMAP sensitive people.

Preparation time: 10minutes

Cooking time: 15minutes

Servings: 4

Ingredients:

2 peaches (halved, pitted and cut into thick slices)

2 nectarines (halved, pitted and cut into thick slices)

2 apricots (halved, pitted and cut into thick slices)

2 plums (halved, pitted and cut into thick slices)

½ cup apple juice

2 tablespoons honey

2 tablespoons unsalted butter (cold, small cubes)

Optional:

1 tablespoon grated ginger

1 tablespoon lemon zest

Directions:

1. Cut the fruits in half, remove the pits and cut them into thick slices. Preheat oven to 400°F.

2. Alternate the fruit slices in a small casserole dish; let it overlap slightly until dish is full. Top with butter and drizzle with honey. Now pour over apple juice, letting it soak. Sprinkle as desired with preferred extra ingredients.

3. Bake fruit 15 minutes or until little char forms on each slice. Turn off the heat and leave in oven for about 5 minutes.

4. Now remove and leave to cool for 10 minutes.

Banana Caramel Ice-Cream
Enjoy this yummy dairy-free ice-cream

Preparation time: 10 minutes

Cooking time: minutes

Servings: 2

Ingredients:

3 frozen bananas, sliced (bananas must be sliced before freezing)

2 heaped tbsp of cashew butter

6 large, soft medjool dates, pitted

2 tbsp canned coconut cream

1 tsp vanilla essence

Directions:

1. Blend the entire ingredients in a blender.

2. Ice cream is ready once the mixture becomes smooth and creamy.

3. Enjoy, sprinkled with a little salt, if desired.

Apple Quinoa Crumble

A healthy version of apple crumble, made even better with quinoa

Preparation time: 5 minutes

Cooking time: 30minutes

Servings: 6

Ingredients:

4 large apples, peeled, cored & diced

1 cup flour

2 cups cooked quinoa

1/2 cashews, walnuts, or pecans, chopped

1/3 cup ground almonds

2 tsp cinnamon

Directions:

1. Preheat oven to 350°F. Oil baking dish or ramekins.

2. Place the apples into it

3. Combine the rest of the ingredients in a bowl and crumble over apples.

4. Bake for 30 minutes until crumble is lightly browned.

Dark Choc Coco Treat
Yummy, and healthy!

Preparation time: 1 hour 30 minutes

Cooking time: 0minutes

Servings: 18

Ingredients:

2 cups desiccated coconut

4 tbsp maple syrup or honey

5 tablespoons coconut oil

1 teaspoon vanilla, alcohol-free

4 oz dark chocolate

Directions:

1. Blend or pulse the coconut until thick. Remove to a bowl and then stir in the maple syrup or honey, coconut oil, and vanilla until thick.

2. Squeeze the mixture in your palm 3 or 4 times; make them into an oval shape, then into 18 half round balls. Now place the coconut balls on cookie sheet (lined with parchment) and place in the refrigerator until firm or for about 30 minutes.

3. Over a double-boiler, melt the chocolate gently until it is smooth and spreadable.

4. Use two forks to roll each coconut ball inside the chocolate until fully covered. Scoop out ball out with the fork and leave the extra chocolate to drip off the fork.

5. Gently place coconut ball that's now covered with chocolate onto the cookie sheet. Sprinkle coconut on top, (to garnish) and chill to harden. Store chocolate in the refrigerator.

SMOOTHIES AND DRINKS

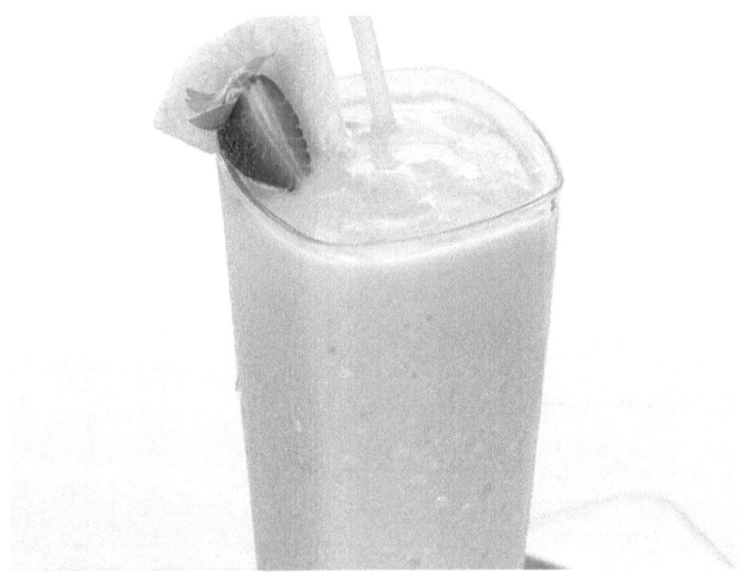

Sunrise Smoothie

Get loads of B vitamins; protein from nut butter; fiber from kale and raspberries; potassium and niacin from banana and oil from flax to help your liver.

Preparation time: 2 minutes

Cooking time: 1minutes

Servings: 1

Ingredients:

1/3 cup of sliced raspberries

1/3 cup of blueberries

1 cup of coconut water

1/2 banana

1/3 cup Greek yogurt, low fat

1/2 cup of chopped kale (chopped)

1/4 cup of cooked and chopped red beets

1 tbsp nut butter

1 teaspoon flax oil

Directions:

1. Blend all the ingredients until smooth. Add distilled to make juicier, if you like.

Licorice Natural Tea

Licorice root is a liver-friendly herb that also addresses several health concerns.

Preparation time: 2 minutes

Cooking time: 1minutes

Servings: 1

Ingredients:

2 1/2 tsp dried licorice root

1/2 cup peppermint leaves, dried &crushed

1/2 cup raw honey

1 cinnamon stick

4 sprigs fresh mint, for taste

6 cups water

Directions:

1. Boil water in a large pot and then add in the licorice and cinnamon, stirring well.

2. Simmer 15 minutes with the pot half partly covered. Remove from heat and then add in the peppermint leaves as well as the other ingredients.

3. Steep10 minutes and then pass it through a strainer. Add the honey, stir well to dissolve.

4. Set aside for 1 hour before drinking.

5. Enjoy hot or iced.

Veggie Juice

Preparation time: 2 minutes

Cooking time: minutes

Servings: 4

Ingredients:

2 celery stalks

3 carrot sticks

1 banana

1 large bunch of broccoli

¼ cup blueberries

5 large organic strawberries

Directions:

1. Add celery, broccoli and carrot sticks to a juicer.

2. Add the fruits to a blender and blend.

3. Add the juicer veggies to the blender and combine well.

Yogurt& Chia Smoothie

Creamy, delicious and satisfying!

Preparation time: 5minutes

Cooking time: minutes

Servings: 1

Ingredients:

2 tablespoons of full fat Greek yogurt

½ cup fresh strawberries

1 tablespoon chia seeds

1 cup nut milk

2 tablespoons of whey protein powder

Directions:

Blend all ingredients until smooth.

Faux-jito Mocktail

While it's not the real deal, this alcohol-free "mocktail" will come in handy at social gatherings and functions. So while others are sipping their cocktail, you're enjoying your mocktail, and maintaining a healthy liver!

Preparation time: 2 minutes

Cooking time: minutes

Servings: 1

Ingredients:

3 lime slices

11 fresh mint leaves

1 tbsp honey

Ice

6 oz soda water or lime- flavored seltzer water

Directions:

1. Place mint leaves and lime inside a tall glass. Stir 1 minute with a spoon to mash content.

2. Add the honey, ice, and then the soda water/seltzer. Stir thoroughly to combine.

3. Garnish drink with lime and mint.

Clean &Fresh Green Juice

A liver-friendly light juice

Preparation time: 5 minutes

Cooking time: minutes

Servings: 1

Ingredients:

1 large green cabbage wedge, washed and cubed

2 small pears, washed, cut in half with cores removed, cubed

1 bunch of romaine leaves

1-inch ginger root, peeled

Directions:

1. Place the washed ingredients in a juicer

2. Pour mixture over ice and enjoy.

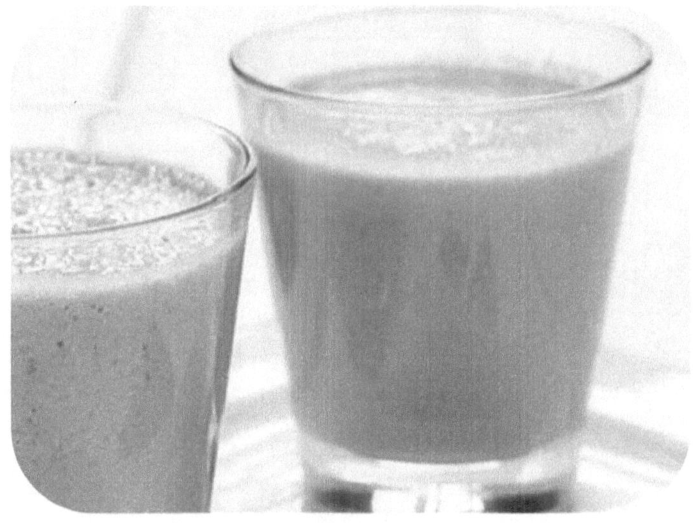

Nourishing Mango Mousse

Preparation time: 2-3 hours

Cooking time: minutes

Servings: 2

Ingredients:

1 mango flesh

1 can full fat coconut milk

½ teaspoon vanilla extract

Directions:

1. Refrigerate coconut milk overnight

2. The next day, blend or process the mango flesh and the vanilla.

3. Bring out the coconut milk from the refrigerator and transfer the solid content only to the blender or processor.

4. Blend all ingredients until mixture is smooth. Remove to serving bowls, cover and chill for at least 2hours before serving.

Liver Cleanse Herbal Tea

Purify your liver and blood by taking this rich herbal tea several times a day.

Preparation time: 5 minutes

Cooking time: 15 minutes

Servings: 1

Ingredients:

1teaspoon red clover blossoms

1 teaspoon nettles

1 teaspoon olive leaf

1/2 teaspoon chickweed

1/2 teaspoon licorice root

1/2 teaspoon fennel seeds

3cups boiling water

Directions:

1. Crush the ingredients and boil 15minutes.

2. Steep, strain and enjoy!

Peppermint Mix Herbal Tea

Keep your liver clean and healthy with this recipe.

Preparation time: 15 minutes

Cooking time: 5 minutes

Servings: 1

Ingredients:

1 handful mint leaves

Juice of 1 lemon

Juice of 1orange

1 lemon, grated

Honey

2 liters of water

Directions:

1. Pour the water into a pot. Add the peppermint leaves and let it boil 5 minutes. Turn heat off heat and let stand.

2. Combine the orange juice, lemon juice, honey and lemon zest in a cup.

3. Get another cup; pour in the peppermint and then add the preparation, mixing well.

4. Drink hot and drink everyday for a week.

Summer Peach Drink

Enjoy the nutritious value of peach.

Preparation time: 10 minutes

Cooking time: minutes

Servings: 1

Ingredients:

4 peaches, peeled & sliced

2½ cups water

Fresh juice of 1 lemon

5 tbsp sweetener of choice

Ice cubes

<u>For Garnish:</u>

Mint leaves

Peach slices

Directions:

1. On medium speed, blend the peach slices. Add lemon juice, water, sugar, and ice cubes.

2. Now blend once more until smooth.

3. Pour the peach juice into glass over the ice.

4. Garnish with mint leaves and peach slices.

SNACKS

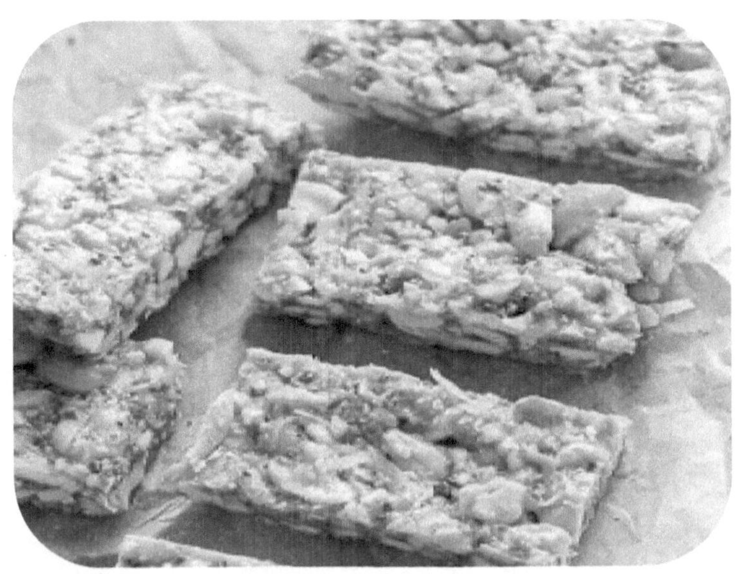

Roasted Cauliflower With Turmeric

An antioxidant-rich side dish you'll enjoy

Preparation time: 10 minutes

Cooking time: 30minutes

Servings: 4

Ingredients:

1 medium head cauliflower, cut into florets

2 tbsp olive oil

2 tsp ground turmeric

Salt and pepper, to taste

Directions:

1. Preheat the oven to 350°Fand then line an oven tray.

2. Brush the florets with olive oil to cover well. Sprinkle with turmeric, salt and pepper.

3. Place in preheated oven and roast until lightly golden.

Apricot Canapés

Impossible to stop at one bite.

Preparation time: 10 minutes

Cooking time: 0 minute

Servings: 16

Ingredients:

2 ounces of pistachios, chopped and shelled

8 teaspoons of blue cheese, crumbled

½ teaspoon of honey

16 dried apricots

Freshly ground pepper

Directions:

1. Top each of the apricots with ½ teaspoon of cheese.

2. Sprinkle the apricots with pistachios.

3. Drizzle honey over it and sprinkle with pepper.

Cashew Coconut Honey Cookies

Since you're watching your sugar consumption, use local honey instead of sugar. This snack recipe contains fiber from old fashioned oats, polyunsaturated fats that helps in digestion and protein to keep you feeling full in- between meals. If you do not like coconut, you can use safflower oil and extra 1/2 cup oat and ground cashews each. Thoroughly vegan!

Preparation time: 5-10 minutes

Cooking time: 20-25minutes

Servings: 24 small cookies

Ingredients:

1/2 cup of local honey

1/2 cup almond flour

1/2 cup cashews, finely ground

1/2 cup coconut oil

1 tbsp lecithin

1 cup unsweetened coconut, shredded

1 cup rolled oats

1/4 whole wheat flour (for gluten-free, substitute extra almond flour)

½ teaspoon of salt

¼ cup almond or coconut milk

Directions:

1. Preheat oven to 350°F.

2. Add the honey, ground cashews, almond flour, lecithin and coconut oil and mix well. Add shredded coconut, whole wheat flour, oats, and salt and mix well to combine. Add milk and stir to make smooth.

3. Use two spoons to drop the cookie dough on a baking sheet lined with parchment paper 2 inches apart. This should provide for about 24 medium-sized cookies.

4. Bake for 20 to 25 minutes, checking for doneness as cooking ends. Remove from oven and leave to cool so that cookies can harden.

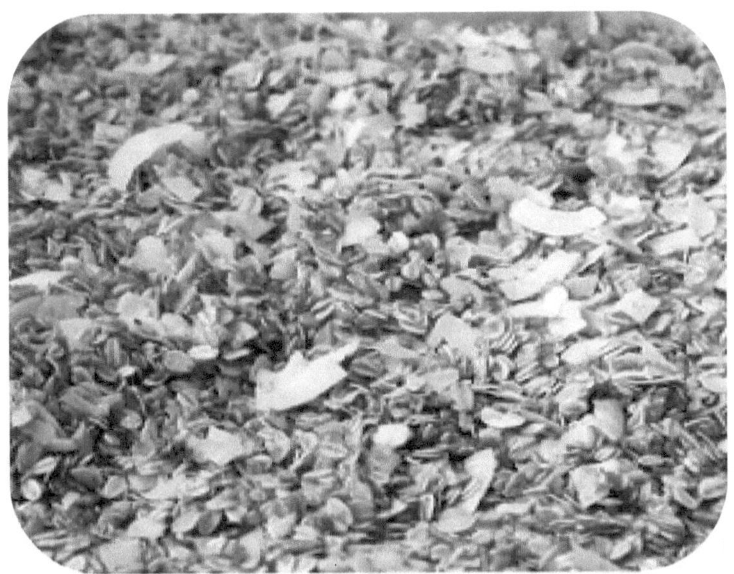

Coconut Granola

Coconut Granola

You can also have this as a dessert, if you desire.

Preparation time: 5 minutes

Cooking time: 21 minutes

Servings: 4-6

Ingredients:

2 cups of no-sugar coconut chips

½ cup of almonds, chopped

½ cup of pecans, chopped

¼ cup of honey

¼ cup coconut oil

¼ cup sunflower seeds

2 tablespoons of chia seeds

1 teaspoon of ground cinnamon

½ teaspoon of ground cloves

Directions:

1. Preheat oven to 350°F.

2. In a small pot on the stove, melt the coconut oil and honey over medium heat.

3. In a large bowl, combine the remaining ingredients. Pour the coconut oil mixture over this and thoroughly mix.

4. Spread the mixture over an oven tray that has been greased or lined.

5. Bake for 15-20 minutes or until it browns lightly.

Date Balls

Those on a vegan and paleo diet will enjoy this easy treat.

Preparation time: 1 hour15 minutes

Cooking time: 0minutes

Servings: 24 small cookies

Ingredients:

2 cups walnuts

1 cup unsweetened coconut, shredded

2 tablespoons coconut oil

2 cups of Medjool dates, soft &pitted

1 tsp vanilla extract

1/2 teaspoon of salt

Directions:

1. Place the coconuts and walnuts in a food processor and process until crumbly. Now add the dates, vanilla, coconut oil, and salt and then process a second time until the batter is a sticky and uniform.

2. Next, form balls by scooping the dough and roll between your hands. Arrange on a lined baking sheet then freeze 1-2 hours before serving, or seal properly before refrigerating.

3. To make a truffle, roll in cocoa powder or shredded coconut before chilling!

Flavorful Italian Quinoa Bites

A delightful treat for your day; however, omit the Asiago, if on a strict low- sodium diet and top off with more zucchini, ¼ cup pine nuts or shaved brussels sprouts.

Preparation time: 5-7 minutes

Cooking time: 20 minutes

Servings: 24 small cookies

Ingredients:

1 cup cooked quinoa

2 large eggs + 1 egg white

½ cup zucchini, shredded

½ cup sun-dried tomatoes, finely chopped

2 tablespoon green onions, chopped

½ cup Asiago cheese, grated

2 tablespoon parsley, chopped

1 tablespoon basil, chopped

Sea salt to taste

Cracked black pepper to taste

Directions:

1. Preheat oven to 350° F.

2. Next, add all the ingredients to a bowl and mix well.

3. Lightly coat a mini muffin pan and spoon the mixture evenly into muffin wells. Bake for 15 to 20 minutes, until the muffins are golden brown. Remove and cool 10 minutes. (If using a regular-sized muffin pan, bake 25 to 30 minutes).

Roasted Cumin Carrots

Maximize all the benefits from carrots with this crunchy snack.

Preparation time: 10 minutes

Cooking time: 30 minutes

Servings: 4

Ingredients:

1 pound of carrots, peeled

1½ tablespoons of ghee

½ tablespoon of ground cumin

¼ teaspoon of salt

½ teaspoon of dried oregano

Directions:

1. Preheat oven to 400°F.

2. Divide the carrots in halves and cut in halves again lengthwise.

3. Arrange the carrot pieces on a greased or lined baking tray.

4. In a small bowl, combine the butter with cumin, salt and oregano. Brush this mixture over the carrots until they are well coated.

5. Roast the carrots for 15-30 minutes or until it is tender and browned lightly

Potato Chips

Microwave made chips with an unforgettable great taste.

Preparation time: 10 minutes

Cooking time: 7 minutes

Servings: 4

Ingredients:

1 1/3 pounds of red or Yukon Gold potatoes, unpeeled, scrubbed and cut into thin 1/8-inch slices.

½ teaspoon of salt

2 teaspoons of extra virgin olive oil

Directions:

1. In a medium bowl, evenly toss the potato slices with the olive oil and salt to coat.

2. With cooking spray, grease a large microwave-proof plate.

3. Arrange the slices of potato on the plate in a single layer.

4. Microwave for 2-3 minutes on high while uncovered. Flip the slices and keep microwaving for 2-4 minutes until the edges begin to brown and turn crispy.

Gingerbread Protein Balls

Preparation time: 10 minutes

Cooking time: minutes

Servings: 4

Ingredients:

1 cup walnuts, roasted

1 cup almonds, roasted

½ cup unsweetened desiccated coconut

1 teaspoon ground cloves

1 tablespoon ground ginger

1tablespoon chia seeds

2 tablespoons honey

Directions:

1. Blend all the ingredients in a food processor and blend until mixture comes together.

2. If dry, add some water.

3. Form mixture into balls, place in a container and refrigerate.

The End